Keto Bread and Keto Desserts Recipe Cookbook

Easy, Low Carb Recipes for Your Ketogenic, Gluten-Free or Paleo Diet that Anyone Can Cook Using Simple Ingredients. All in 1 - Keto Bread, Keto Fat Bombs, No Carb Keto Cookies and Keto Snacks and Treats, Keto Ice Cream, Pudding, Mousse

This document is geared towards providing exact and reliable information in regards to the topic and issue covered. The publication is sold with the idea that the publisher is not required to render an accounting, officially permitted, or otherwise, qualified services. If advice is necessary, legal or professional, a practised individual in the profession should be ordered.

From a Declaration of Principles which was accepted and approved equally by a Committee of the American Bar Association and a Committee of Publishers and Associations.

Table of Contents

Chapter 1. «Everything You Need to Know About the Ketogenic Diet»

Thanks to the increasing demand for healthy diets and lifestyles, the ketogenic diet has taken center stage. Also known as a low-carb, high-fat meal plan, the keto diet restricts the intake of carbohydrates while promoting healthy fats. Usually, confectioneries and baked goods, snacks, and desserts contain the most carbs since they're predominantly made of sugars and flour. They're also the types of foods that people typically break their diets to eat.

Therefore, this cookbook is full of keto versions of snacks, desserts, and other treats that would normally be forbidden on the low-carb diet. Along with the recipes, you'll also get the ultimate ketogenic guidelines that explain basic information on ketogenic-friendly flours and sweeteners.

The Ketogenic Diet: Concept and Benefits

After years of research and experimentation, scientists and nutritionists worked together to come up with an efficient formula that would not only treat mental illnesses like Alzheimer's and Parkinson's disease but also had a broad impact over general human health. This diet plan created miraculous effects like reducing obesity and controlling insulin in diabetic patients. It eventually came to be known as the ketogenic diet.

The word "keto" comes from the process of ketosis—a physical reaction in the body that this diet produces when followed properly. Ketosis is a metabolic process that uses stored fats for energy when there isn't enough glucose in the body to use. This makes it ideal for losing weight while also debunking the myth that fats in food are linked to weight gain. With this diet, the human body can harness more energy from food while producing ketones (a product of ketosis) which detoxify the blood and mind.

In order for any of this to work properly, you have to cut your carb intake using ketogenic carb recommendations. The main carb restriction states that your intake per meal should be no more than 13 grams of carbs. It also requires you go to embrace high-fat foods instead. Combine this with regular exercise and you can see the weight loss results you desire. To reduce carbohydrates in your diet, you'll need to remove or limit high-carb ingredients like all grains, lentils, legumes, potatoes, yams, yellow squash, sugars, honey, high-carb fruits, syrups, and the like. You can either avoid them or replace them with low-carb alternatives.

If a person successfully follows the ketogenic diet for about three to four weeks, they can witness marked changes in their physical and mental health. An obese person can lose about two to three pounds in this time period and a diabetic patient can experience stable insulin levels. People with mental ailments can feel better control over their nerves and emotions, too. Following this diet and lifestyle over a long period of time can even decrease your risk of cancer and complicated cardiac diseases. Cholesterol levels can also be maintained following the ketogenic diet.

What to Eat and What Not to Eat on a Ketogenic Diet

Eating foods high in fat and low in carbs may sound simple but it is more difficult to practically implement this idea if you are not familiar with the basics of nutrients. To help you, here is some brief insight regarding all the foods that are restricted and allowed on the ketogenic diet.

First, here are keto-friendly foods to add to your menu:

1. All dairy and plant fats are ideal for the ketogenic diet. This includes all forms of plants, oils, butter, ghee, cream, and cheese.

2. All dairy products except milk are suitable for a ketogenic diet. Since milk contains high traces of carbohydrates, it is restricted. When milk is

10

processed to produce yogurt, cream cheese, cream, and other cheeses, the carbs are broken down making them keto-friendly.

3. All vegetables low in carbs are allowed on the ketogenic diet including all greens, above-ground vegetables, onions, garlic, ginger, and similar vegetables.

4. While most fruits should be limited or avoided, all berries and similar fruits are keto-friendly.

5. All sugar-free chocolates, sauces, and syrups are safe to use on a ketogenic diet.

6. Ketogenic sugar substitutes are allowed.

7. Nut-based milk like almond milk, coconut milk, hemp milk, soy milk, etc. are also low- carb and, thus, safe to use.

While knowing what you can eat is great, knowing what not to eat on the ketogenic diet should be your major focus. First, get into the habit of reading labels and nutrition facts for every food you buy to make yourself comfortable with looking for carbs in food. You can't expect to control your carb intake without reading labels. Then, follow this list of high-carb ingredients while grocery shopping and keep them out of your kitchen.

1. All grains, legumes, lentils, and beans are rich in carbohydrates, so avoid them in any form. Rice, wheat, barley, oats, chickpeas, kidney beans, corn, sorghum, etc. are all a part of this category, too.

2. Potatoes, yams, beets, yellow squash, and similar vegetables are considered starchy vegetables, and are high in carbs and should be avoided.

3. Apples, bananas, peaches, pears, melons, watermelons, mangoes, pineapples, and similar fruits are all carb-rich and are not allowed on the ketogenic diet.

4. Any amount of animal milk is restricted. Replace that with nut-based milks.

5. Flours from grains and lentils like wheat flour, all-purpose flours, and chickpea flour should be avoided and replaced with nut-based gluten-free flours.

6. White sugars, brown sugars, sugary syrups and beverages, maple syrups, honey, and dates are all forbidden on a ketogenic diet. Replace them with ketogenic sweeteners to add sweetness.

7. All processed foods with traces of carbohydrates need to be avoided.

Types of Gluten-Free Ketogenic Flours

Flours are an important component of all baked desserts, breads, and confectioneries so they can't be altogether avoided. Since grain- and lentil-based flours are not suitable for the ketogenic diet, look to other gluten-free options to produce the same products with a lower carb content. Those include:

1. Almond Flour

This flour comes from almonds finely ground into a powder and is used for baking low-carb breads and desserts. There are two varieties available for almond flour: blanched and unblanched almond flour. The former is from blanched and peeled almonds whereas the latter is obtained from grinding the raw nuts. Blanched flour is more refined and mostly used for making bread and other desserts. Unblanched flour is less refined and not purely off-white in color. Instead, it has mixed shades of white and brown. Blanched flour is completely off-white in color with a fluffier texture.

2. Almond Meal

Almond meal is not the same as almond flour. Meal is coarser and not ideal for every bread, dessert or confectionery. Instead, it's only used when you need a crumbly texture for a recipe. Keep this differentiation in your mind when choosing ingredients; don't substitute one for the other.

3. Coconut Flour

Coconut flour, as the name indicates, comes from the dehydrated white flesh of a coconut. It is so finely ground that it turns into flour and gives a nice texture and taste to recipes. When it comes to texture, coconut flour is not exactly like wheat flour; it is denser and can soak up more moisture than wheat flour. Due to this, extra water or liquid needs to be added to give coconut flour the same texture batters or doughs. This flour can also make lots of clumps in a batter; use a good beater or whisk your mixtures well with a fork to break up any clumps.

4. Ground Flaxseed

Flaxseeds are a rich source of healthy fats, vitamins, minerals, and antioxidants making them quite beneficial for digestion and heart health. Flaxseed flour and meal can both be used in the ketogenic diet. Flaxseed bread, muffins, and cookie recipes are in this book to give you a simple idea on how to use this super nourishing seed flour or meal. Like almond meal, flaxseed meal is coarser than the ground flour so take that into account when following recipes. Processed flaxseed flour is available at most grocery stores.

5. Psyllium Husk Powder

This commonly known husk is obtained from the seeds of Plantago ovata. Basically, it is a good soluble fiber supplement. Available in both powder and husk form, this supplement is also good for the ketogenic diet. The powder is suitable to use in several ketogenic breads, desserts, and confectioneries as it has a light and airy touch that gives food a fluffy and soft texture.

Chapter 2 «Guide to Low Carb Sweeteners Used in Baking»

Sweeteners play an important part in building the right balance of flavor in baked desserts. It's not just cakes or cookies that need sweeteners. Almost all desserts from custard to mousses, fat bombs, and ice creams need a good sweetener. Since sugar is not an option on a ketogenic diet, you should rely on other low-carb substitutes that are specially manufactured for such a diet. Those substitutes mainly include:

- Stevia

Stevia is the strongest of all and tastes 200 times sweeter than ordinary white sugar. It should be used in very small amounts. It is available in a range of varieties including powdered and liquid form. Be extra careful while adding this intense sweetener to your recipes. One cup of sugar can be replaced with a teaspoon of stevia powder to get the same sweetness. Stevia is completely natural and comes from the stevia plant so it doesn't have any negative effects on your health.

- Erythritol

Erythritol is a sugar alcohol. These kinds of substances do taste sweet, but don't contain many calories and carbohydrates. Since erythritol has a sweetness level close to that of ordinary sugar, it is more commonly used for ketogenic desserts. As you'll see on the chart, its conversion is simpler than stevia, too. Another plus point for erythritol is that it contains an extremely low amount of calories. Where one gram of sugar has around four calories, the same amount of erythritol contains only 0.24 calories. Erythritol is available in a powdered form and can be used easily in baking.

- Xylitol

Xylitol is also a naturally occurring sugar alcohol that can be used to sweeten ketogenic desserts. Where other sweeteners discussed above are used for cakes and cookies, xylitol is best suited for ketogenic candies and gums. This is probably due to the taste and texture of this natural sweetener. It comes from plants like fruits and vegetables. Due to its health benefits and curing powers, it is also added to medicines and mints to keep the gums and breath fresh. It is not only low in carbohydrates, but it contains few calories and ranks very low on the glycemic index.

- Sorbitol

Another sugar alcohol, sorbitol is found in several fruits and it is also present in corn syrup. It is also known as a nutritive sweetener since it can provide as many as 2.6 kcals per gram. Like xylitol, it is also great for sweets, candies, mints, gummies, and bites. It has other medicinal properties that make it good for older people. Whether it's keto or any other diet, the use of this sweetener is always good for your health. It is 60 percent the sweetness of sugar so 1 cup of sugar can be replace with 1 ¼ cups of sorbitol.

• Miscellaneous Sweeteners

Swerve is another ketogenic sweetener not only used in baking, but also for ice creams, mousses, fat bombs, and other desserts. Since Swerve is available in all forms including powder, granulated, white, and even brown making it perfect for adding texture to different baked items. Monk fruit sweetener is another good option to sweeten your ketogenic desserts and to give them nice taste and texture.

Conversion Chart

SUGAR	1 TSP	1 TBSP	1/4 CUP	1/3 CUP	1/2 CUP	1 CUP
Erythritol	1 1/4 tsp	1 Tbsp + 1 tsp	1/3 cup	1/3 cup + 2 Tbsp	2/3 cup	1 1/3 cup
Xylitol	1 tsp	1 Tbsp	1/4 cup	1/3 cup	1/2 cup	1 cup

Swerve	1 tsp	1 Tbsp	1/4 cup	1/3 cup	1/2 cup	1 cup
Stevia	-	-	3/16 tsp	1/4 tsp	3/8 tsp	3/4 tsp
Liquid Stevia	3/8 tsp	3/8 tsp	1 1/2 tsp	2 tsp	3 tsp	2 Tbsp
Sukrin:	1 tsp	1 Tbsp	1/4 cup	1/3 cup	1/2 cup	1 cup

Sugar Alcohols Glycemic Index

Sugar alcohols are neither sugars nor alcohols; they are naturally existing compounds that are sweet in taste without being high in carbs or calories. They are considered dietary fibers due to their chemical composition.

The glycemic index of a food is used to determine if it's suitable for the ketogenic diet. Since sugar has the highest glycemic value 60, all other sweeteners are compared to this value to calculate their glycemic values. All sugar alcohols have very low glycemic values and, therefore, are keto-friendly. Here is a list of commonly used sugar alcohols along with their glycemic values:

Sugar Alcohols	Glycemic Index
Xylitol	12
Glycerol	5

Sorbitol	4
Lactitol	3
Isomalt	2
Mannitol	2
Erythritol	1

Chapter 3 Keto Bread Recipes

Keto Pumpkin Bread

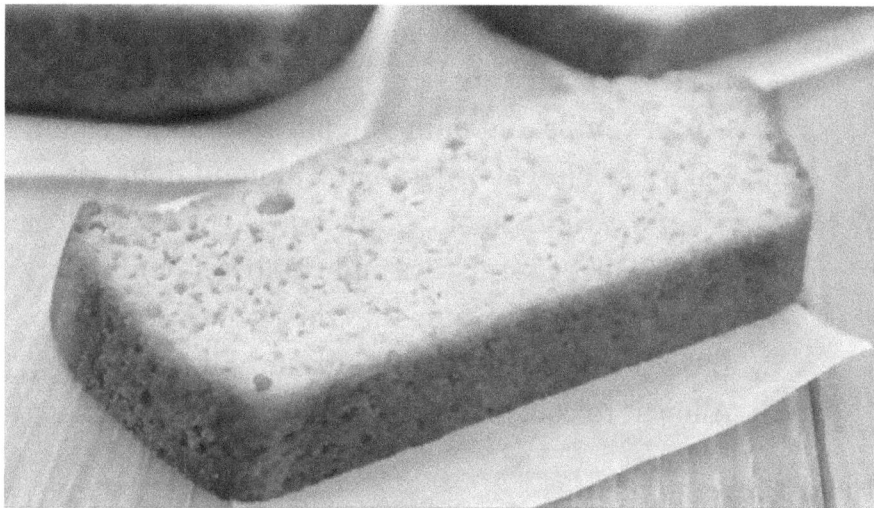

Ingredients:
- 1/½ cup butter, softened
- 2/3 cup erythritol sweetener
- 4 large eggs
- ¾ cup pumpkin puree, canned
- 1 tsp vanilla extract
- 1 ½ cup almond flour
- ½ cup coconut flour
- 4 tsp baking powder
- 1 tsp cinnamon
- ½ tsp nutmeg
- ¼ tsp ginger
- 8 tsp cloves
- ½ tsp salt

How to Prepare:

1. Preheat your oven to 350 degrees F and grease a 9x5-inch piece of wax paper and fit into a loaf pan.
2. Beat butter with sweetener in a mixer until foamy.
3. Whisk in eggs one by one while continuously beating the mixture.
4. Stir in vanilla and pumpkin puree then mix again.
5. Take a separate bowl and mix almond flour with other dry ingredients in this bowl.
6. Stir in wet eggs mixture and combine them well.
7. Pour this batter evenly into the prepared loaf pan.
8. Bake the bread for 55 minutes until it is done.
9. Allow it to cool on a wire rack then slice to serve.

Prep Time: 5 minutes
Cooking Time: 55 minutes
Total Time: 60 minutes
Servings: 10 slices

Nutritional Values:

- *Calories 165*
- *Total Fat 14 g*
- *Saturated Fat 7 g*
- *Cholesterol 632 mg*
- *Sodium 497 mg*
- *Total Carbs 6 g*
- *Fiber 3 g*
- *Sugar 1 g*
- *Protein 5 g*

Low Carb Blueberry Bread

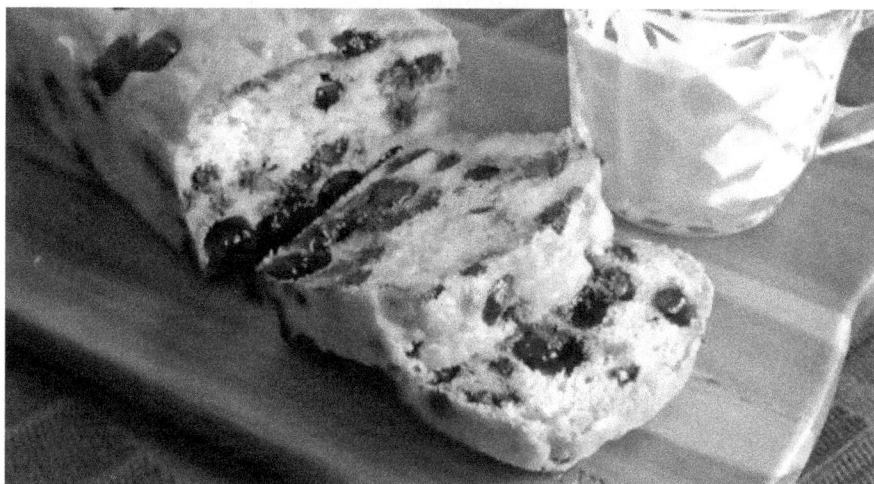

Ingredients:

- ½ cup almond butter
- ¼ cup butter
- ½ cup almond flour
- ½ tsp salt
- 2 tsp baking powder
- ½ cup almond milk, unsweetened
- 5 eggs, beaten
- ½ cup blueberries

How to Prepare:
1. Preheat your oven to 350 degrees F.
2. Melt the butter in a bowl in the microwave then mix well.

3. Whisk almond butter with salt, baking powder, and almond flour in a suitable bowl.
4. Stir in almond milk and egg while beating the mixture.
5. Fold in berries and mix gently.
6. Layer a loaf pan with wax paper and grease it lightly with cooking oil.
7. Pour the blueberry batter into the loaf pan.
8. Bake for 45 minutes.
9. Allow it to cool on a wire rack for 30 minutes.
10. Slice and serve.

Prep Time: 5 minutes
Cooking Time: 45 minutes
Total Time: 50 minutes
Servings: 12 slices

Nutritional Values:
- *Calories 107*
- *Total Fat 9.3 g*
- *Saturated Fat 4.8 g*
- *Cholesterol 77 mg*
- *Sodium 135 mg*
- *Total Carbs 2.6 g*
- *Fiber 0.8 g*
- *Sugar 9.9 g*
- *Protein 3.9 g*

Cinnamon Almond Flour Bread

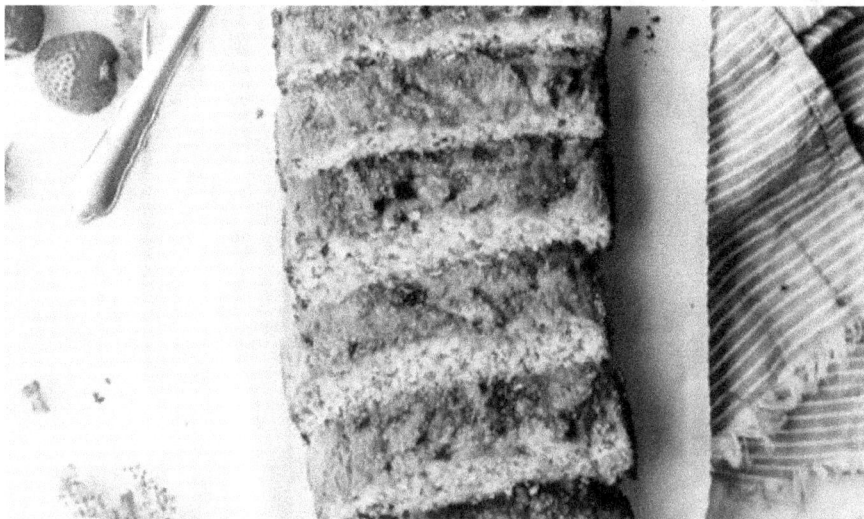

Ingredients:

- 2 cups fine, blanched almond flour
- 2 tbsp coconut flour
- ½ tsp sea salt
- 1 tsp baking soda
- ¼ cup flaxseed meal
- 5 eggs + 1 egg white
- 1 ½ tsp apple cider vinegar
- 2 tbsp maple syrup or honey
- 2–3 tbsp clarified butter (melted)
- 1 tbsp cinnamon + extra for topping

How to Prepare:

1. Preheat your oven to 350 degrees F. Layer an 8x4-inch loaf pan with wax paper.

2. In a bowl, mix coconut flour, baking soda, salt, almond flour, flaxseed meal, and ½ tbsp cinnamon.
3. Beat the egg white and eggs separately then stir in maple syrup, vinegar, and 1 tbsp butter.
4. Stir in coconut flour mixture and combine until smooth.
5. Spread the batter evenly in the loaf pan.
6. Bake the bread for 35 minutes at 350 degrees F.
7. Allow it to cool on a wire rack.
8. Mix 1 tbsp melted butter with ½ tbsp cinnamon and brush this butter over the bread.
9. Serve.

Prep Time: 15 minutes
Cooking Time: 35 minutes
Total Time: 50 minutes
Servings: 12 slices

Nutritional Values:
- *Calories 106*
- *Total Fat 5.9 g*
- *Saturated Fat 1.5 g*
- *Cholesterol 3 mg*
- *Sodium 313 mg*
- *Total Carbs 8.5 g*
- *Fiber 3.2 g*
- *Sugar 3.7 g*
- *Protein 4.7 g*

Cranberry Bread

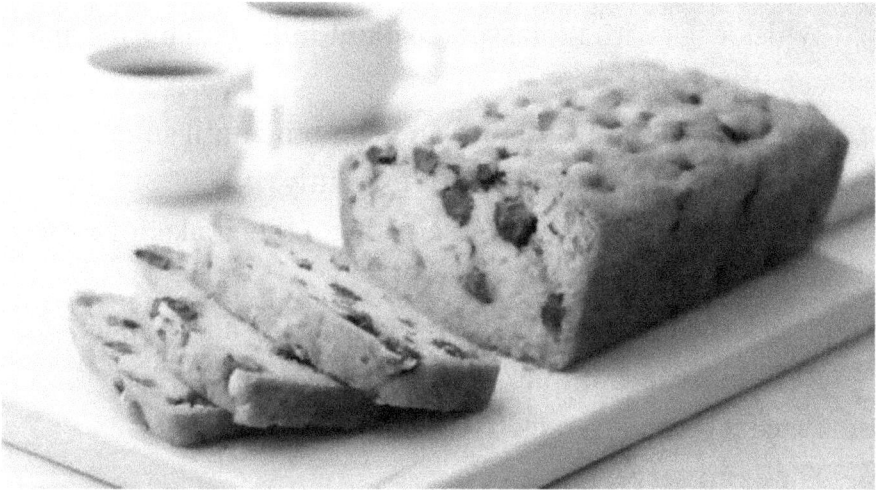

Ingredients:

- 2 cups almond flour
- ½ cup powdered erythritol
- ½ tsp stevia powder
- 1 ½ tsp baking powder
- ½ tsp baking soda
- 1 tsp salt
- 4 tbsp unsalted butter, melted
- 1 tsp blackstrap molasses
- 4 large eggs
- ½ cup coconut milk
- 1 12-oz bag cranberries

How to Prepare:

1. Preheat your oven to 350 degrees F. Grease a 9x5-inch loaf pan with cooking oil.

2. Mix flour with baking powder, baking soda, stevia, salt, and erythritol in a large bowl.
3. Whisk eggs with molasses, coconut milk, and butter in a separate bowl.
4. Stir in sweet flour mixture and combine until smooth.
5. Fold in the cranberries and mix gently.
6. Spread this berry batter in a loaf pan then bake for 1 hour and 15 minutes.
7. Check the bread after 1 hour by inserting a toothpick. Bake more if toothpick doesn't come out clean.
8. Place it on a wire rack to cool down.
9. Slice and serve.

Prep Time: 10 minutes
Cooking Time: 1 hour & 15 minutes
Total Time: 1 hour & 25 minutes
Servings: 12 slices

Nutritional Values:
- *Calories 172*
- *Total Fat 10.7 g*
- *Saturated Fat 7.4 g*
- *Cholesterol 62 mg*
- *Sodium 121 mg*
- *Total Carbs 4.9 g*
- *Fiber 0.6 g*
- *Sugar 17.3 g*
- *Protein 4 g*

Coconut Bread

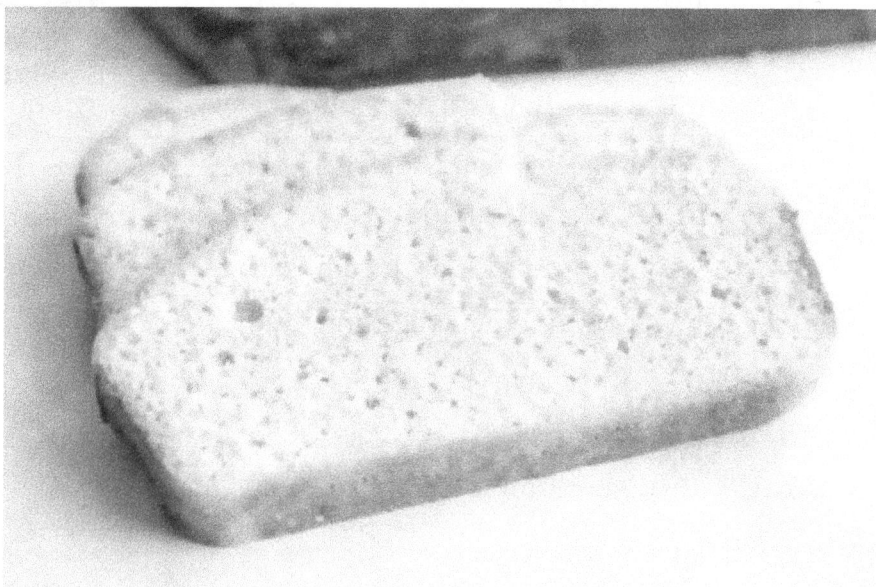

Ingredients:

- ½ cup coconut flour
- ¼ tsp salt
- ¼ tsp baking soda
- 6 eggs
- ¼ cup coconut oil, melted
- ¼ unsweetened almond milk

How to Prepare:

1. Preheat your oven to 350 degrees F. Layer an 8x4-inch loaf pan with wax paper.

2. Mix coconut flour with salt and baking soda in a suitable bowl.
3. Whisk eggs with oil and milk in a separate bowl.
4. Stir coconut flour mixture into the egg mixture and combine until smooth.
5. Spread this bread batter in the loaf pan.
6. Bake it for 50 minutes until it is done.
7. Allow it to cool then slice and enjoy.

Prep Time: 15 minutes
Cooking Time: 50 minutes
Total Time: 65 minutes
Servings: 10 slices

Nutritional Values:

- *Calories 192*
- *Total Fat 11.8 g*
- *Saturated Fat 3.9 g*
- *Cholesterol 135 mg*
- *Sodium 187 mg*
- *Total Carbs 4.1 g*
- *Fiber 0.1g*
- *Sugar 2.1 g*
- *Protein 5.9 g*

Cloud Bread

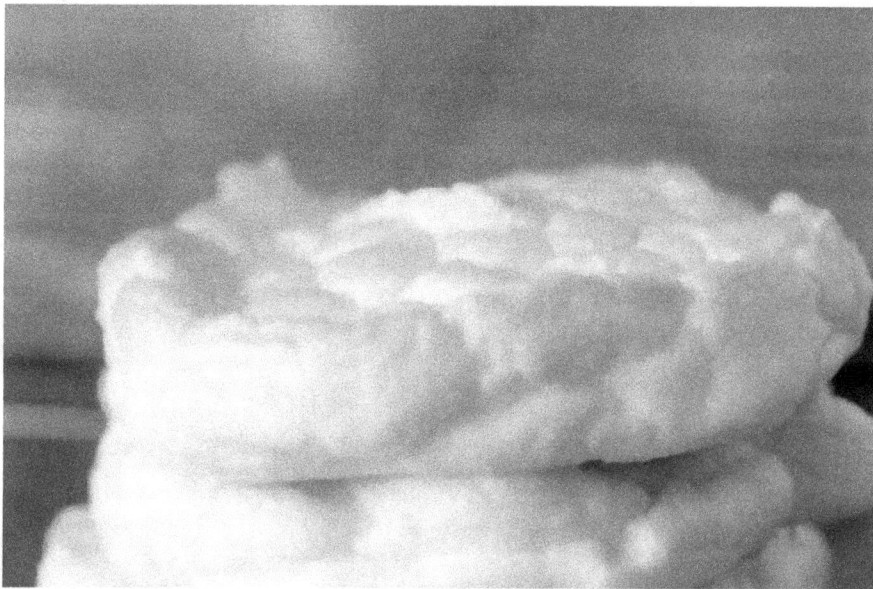

Ingredients:

- 3 eggs
- 3 tbsp coconut cream
- ½ tsp baking powder
- 1 Pinch sea salt
- 1 pinch black pepper
- 1 pinch dried rosemary

How to Prepare:

1. Preheat your oven to 325 degrees F. Layer a baking sheet with wax paper.
2. Separate the egg yolks from the whites then add the yolks to a bowl with the coconut cream.
3. Beat well with a hand mixer until fluffy.

4. Whisk egg whites with baking powder in a separate bowl using the hand mixer.
5. Beat it until thick and foamy.
6. Add the egg yolk mixture to the whites and mix well.
7. Drop the batter onto the baking sheet spoon by spoon to get 4-inch separate circles.
8. Bake them for 25 minutes in the oven.
9. Enjoy.

Prep Time: 15 minutes
Cooking Time: 25 minutes
Total Time: 40 minutes
Servings: 4

Nutritional Values:

- *Calories 233*
- *Total Fat 20.2 g*
- *Saturated Fat 4.4 g*
- *Cholesterol 120 mg*
- *Sodium 76 mg*
- *Total Carbs 3.5 g*
- *Fiber 0.9 g*
- *Sugar 1.4 g*
- *Protein 1.9 g*

Garlic & Herb Focaccia

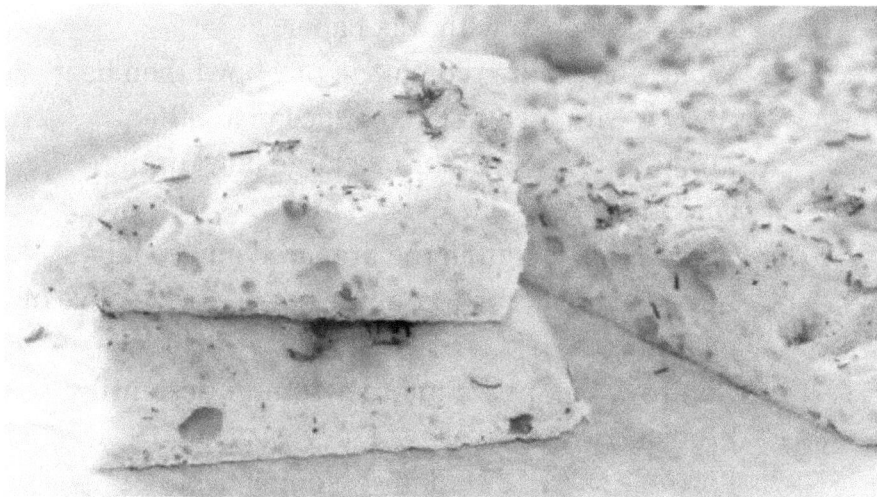

Ingredients:

Dry Ingredients

- 1 cup almond flour
- ¼ cup coconut flour
- ½ tsp xanthan gum
- 1 tsp garlic powder
- 1 tsp flaky salt
- ½ tsp baking soda
- ½ tsp baking powder
- Italian seasonings, to garnish
- Salt flakes, to garnish

Wet Ingredients

- 2 eggs
- 1 tbsp lemon juice
- 2 tsp olive oil + 2 tbsp olive oil to drizzle

How to Prepare:

1. Preheat your oven to 350 degrees F. Layer an 8-inch baking pan with wax paper.
2. Whisk the dry ingredients in one bowl then beat the egg with oil and lemon juice in another.
3. Mix these two together in a large bowl until smooth.
4. Spread this dough in the prepared pan evenly.
5. Bake the bread for 10 minutes then drizzle olive oil over it.
6. Continue baking for another 10 minutes until brown.
7. Sprinkle salt and Italian seasoning over it.
8. Enjoy.

Prep Time: 10 minutes
Cooking Time: 20 minutes
Total Time: 30 minutes
Servings: 8

Nutritional Values:

- *Calories 121*
- *Total Fat 12.2 g*
- *Saturated Fat 2.4 g*
- *Cholesterol 110 mg*
- *Sodium 276 mg*
- *Total Carbs 3 g*
- *Fiber 0.9 g*
- *Sugar 1.4 g*
- *Protein 1.8 g*

Cauliflower Tartar Bread

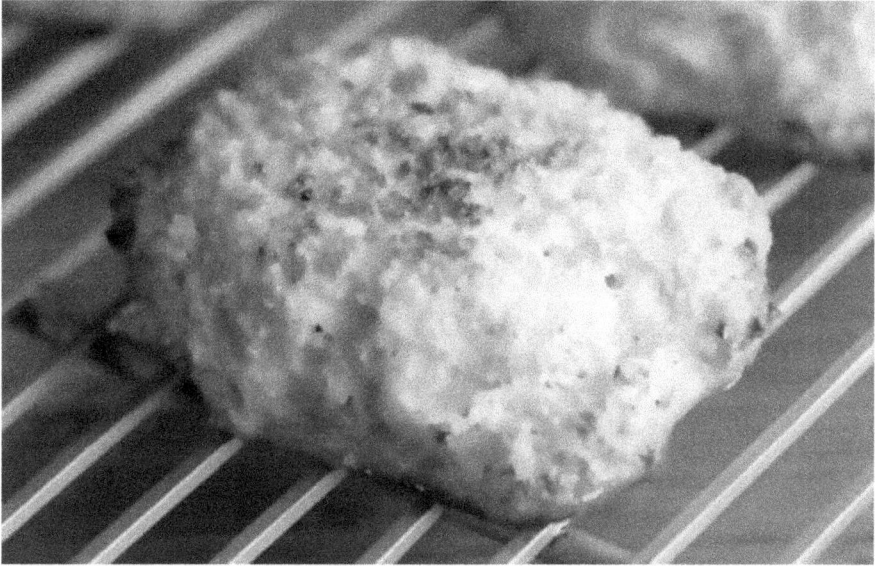

Ingredients:

- 3 cup cauliflower rice
- 10 large eggs, yolks and egg whites separated
- ¼ tsp cream of tartar
- 1 ¼ cup coconut flour
- 1 ½ tbsp gluten-free baking powder
- 1 tsp sea salt
- 6 tbsp butter
- 6 cloves garlic, minced
- 1 tbsp fresh rosemary, chopped
- 1 tbsp fresh parsley, chopped

How to Prepare:

1. Preheat your oven to 350 degrees F. Layer a 9x5-inch pan with wax paper.
2. Place the cauliflower rice in a suitable bowl and then cover it with plastic wrap.
3. Heat it for 4 minutes in the microwave. Heat more if the cauliflower isn't soft enough.
4. Place the cauliflower rice in a kitchen towel and squeeze it to drain excess water.
5. Transfer drained cauliflower rice to a food processor.
6. Add coconut flour, sea salt, baking powder, butter, egg yolks, and garlic. Blend until crumbly.
7. Beat egg whites with cream of tartar in a bowl until foamy.
8. Add the egg whites mixture to the cauliflower mixture and stir well with a spatula.
9. Fold in rosemary and parsley.
10. Spread this batter in the prepared baking pan evenly.
11. Bake it for 50 minutes until golden then allow it to cool.
12. Slice and serve.

Prep Time: 15 minutes
Cooking Time: 50 minutes

Total Time: 65 minutes

Servings: 6

Nutritional Values:

- Calories 104
- Total Fat 8.9 g
- Saturated Fat 4.5 g
- Cholesterol 57 mg
- Sodium 340 mg
- Total Carbs 4.7 g
- Fiber 1.2 g
- Sugar 1.3 g
- Protein 3.3g

Buttery Skillet Flatbread

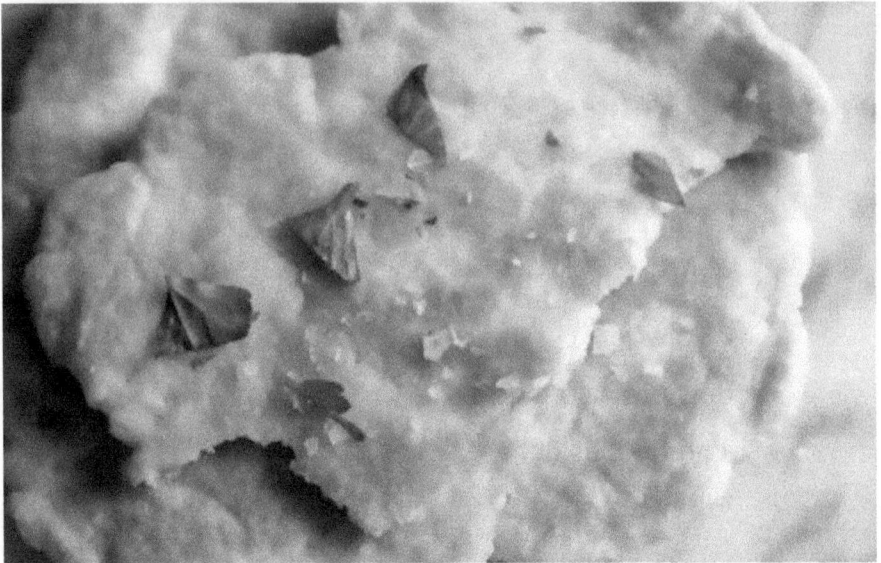

Ingredients:

- 1 cup almond flour
- 2 tbsp coconut flour
- 2 tsp xanthan gum
- ½ tsp baking powder
- ½ tsp salt
- 1 whole egg + 1 egg white
- 1 tbsp water (if needed)
- 1 tbsp oil, for frying
- 1 tbsp melted butter, for brushing

How to prepare:

1. Mix xanthan gum with flours, salt, and baking powder in a suitable bowl.

2. Beat egg and egg white in a separate bowl then stir in the flour mixture.
3. Mix well until smooth. Add a tablespoon of water if the dough is too thick.
4. Divide the dough into 4 equal portions and then spread them into ¼-inch thick rounds.
5. Place a large skillet over medium heat and heat oil.
6. Add one round in the skillet and cook for 1 minute per side.
7. Cook the remaining rounds in the skillet and place them in a platter when done.
8. Mix butter with salt and parsley.
9. Brush butter over the bread and enjoy.

Prep Time: 10 minutes
Cooking Time: 10 minutes
Total Time: 20 minutes
Servings: 4

Nutritional Values:
- *Calories 272*
- *Total Fat 18 g*
- *Saturated Fat 5 g*
- *Cholesterol 6.1 mg*
- *Sodium 3 mg*
- *Total Carbs 4 g*
- *Fiber 3 g*
- *Sugar 4 g*
- *Protein 0.4 g*

Zucchini Bread with Walnuts

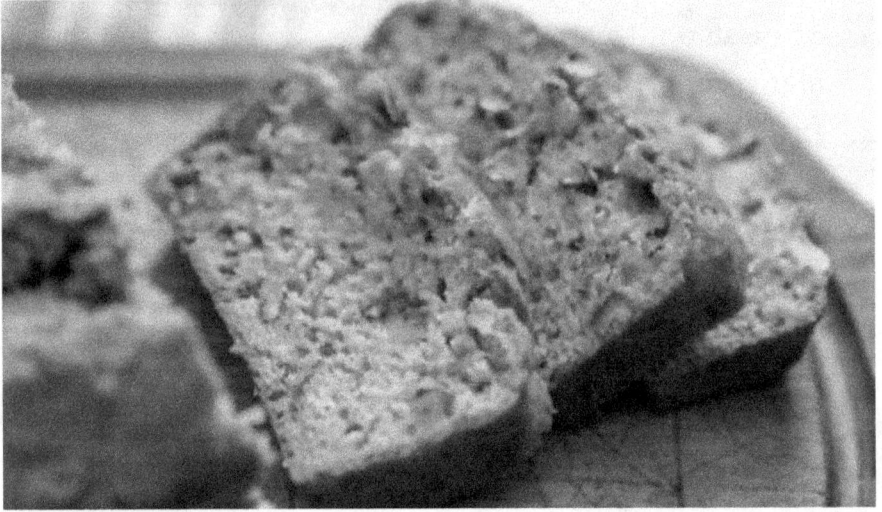

Ingredients:
- 3 large eggs
- ½ cup olive oil
- 1 tsp vanilla extract
- 2 ½ cups almond flour
- 1 ½ cups erythritol
- ½ tsp salt
- 1 ½ tsp baking powder
- ½ tsp nutmeg
- 1 tsp ground cinnamon
- ¼ tsp ground ginger
- 1 cup grated zucchini
- ½ cup chopped walnuts

How to Prepare:
1. Preheat your oven to 350 degrees F.

2. Beat eggs with vanilla extract and oil in a mixer.
3. Whisk almond flour with baking powder, salt, erythritol, ginger, cinnamon, and nutmeg in a separate bowl.
4. Stir in egg mixture and mix well until incorporated.
5. Place zucchini in cheesecloth and squeeze the excess water out of it.
6. Add this zucchini to the egg and flour mixture then mix well.
7. Grease a 9x5-inch loaf pan with cooking oil and spread the batter in the pan.
8. Sprinkle chopped walnuts on top then bake for 70 minutes at 350 degrees F.
9. Slice and serve.

Prep Time: 15 minutes
Cooking Time: 70 minutes
Total Time: 85 minutes
Servings: 8

Nutritional Values:
- *Calories 201*
- *Total Fat 12.2 g*
- *Saturated Fat 2.4 g*
- *Cholesterol 110 mg*
- *Sodium 276 mg*
- *Total Carbs 4.3 g*
- *Fiber 0.9 g*
- *Sugar 1.4 g*
- *Protein 8.8 g*

Sesame Keto Bread

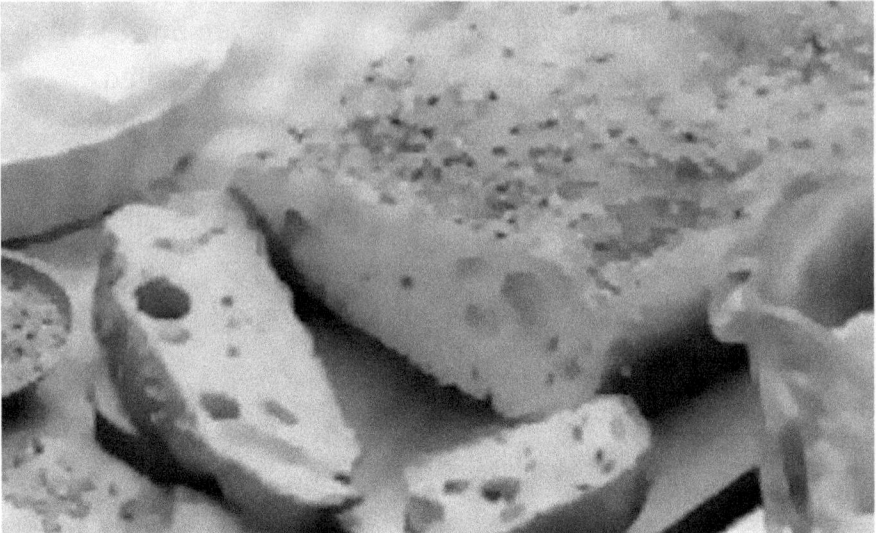

Ingredients:

- 5 tbsp ground psyllium husk powder
- 1¼ cup almond flour
- 2 tsp baking powder
- 1 tsp sea salt
- 1 cup water
- 2 tsp cider vinegar
- 3 egg whites
- 2 tbsp sesame seeds (optional)

How to Prepare:

1. Preheat your oven to 350 degrees F.
2. Pour water in a pot then boil it.
3. Meanwhile, mix the dry ingredients for the batter in a suitable bowl.

4. Beat egg whites and vinegar in a separate bowl then stir in boiled water and dry mixture.
5. Beat it for 30 seconds with a hand mixer until smooth.
6. Make six rolls out of this dough then place them on a greased baking sheet.
7. Sprinkle sesame seeds over the rolls and press them gently.
8. Bake them for 60 minutes on the lower rack and garnish as desired.
9. Enjoy.

Prep Time: 5 minutes
Cooking Time: 60 minutes
Total Time: 65 minutes
Servings: 8

Nutritional Values:
- *Calories 151*
- *Total Fat 12.2 g*
- *Saturated Fat 2.4 g*
- *Cholesterol 110 mg*
- *Sodium 276 mg*
- *Total Carbs 3.2 g*
- *Fiber 1.9 g*
- *Sugar 0.4 g*
- *Protein 8.8 g*

Keto Ramekin Bread

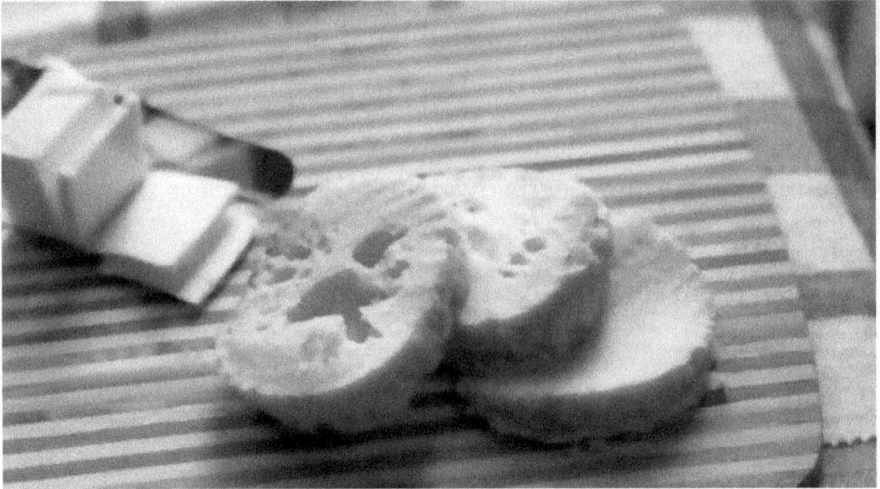

Ingredients:

- 1 egg
- 1 tbsp butter
- 3 tbsp almond flour
- ½ tsp baking powder

How to Prepare:

1. Add all the ingredients for keto bread to a small bowl.
2. Pour this batter into a greased ramekin then place in the microwave.
3. Let it cook for 90 seconds on high heat then remove the bread from the ramekin.

4. Cut it in half then add the halves to a greased skillet.
5. Sear the bread in the skillet over medium heat until golden brown on all sides.
6. Enjoy.

Prep Time: 5 minutes
Cooking Time: 3 minutes
Total Time: 8 minutes
Servings: 1

Nutritional Values:

- *Calories 173*
- *Total Fat 16.2 g*
- *Saturated Fat 9.8 g*
- *Cholesterol 100 mg*
- *Total Carbs 9.4 g*
- *Sugar 0.2 g*
- *Fiber 1 g*
- *Sodium 42 mg*
- *Protein 3.3 g*

Chewy Poppyseed Bread

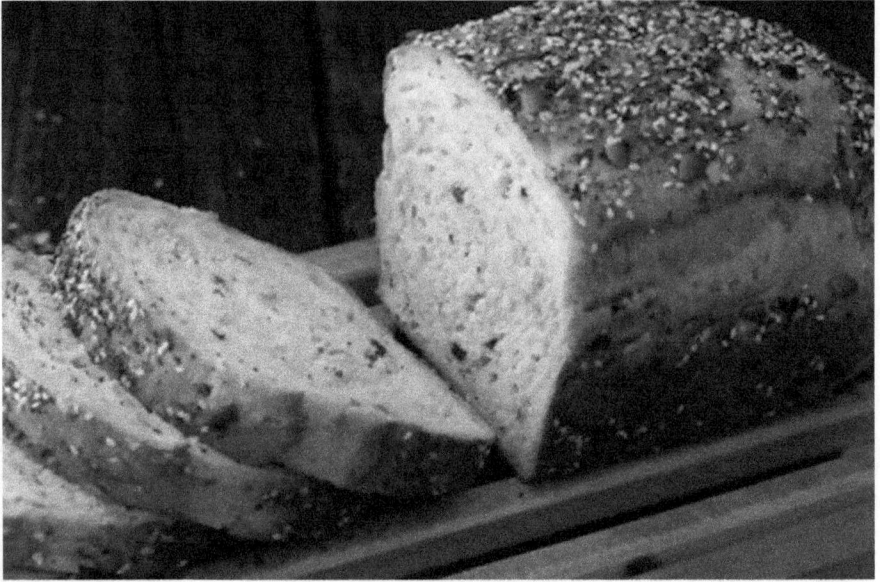

Ingredients:

- ½ cup coconut flour
- 2 tsp baking powder
- ¾ tsp xanthan gum
- 12 oz pre-shredded mozzarella
- 2 large eggs

Topping

- 1 tsp sesame seeds
- 1 tsp poppyseed
- 1 tsp dried, minced onion

- ½ tsp coarse salt
- 1 tbsp butter melted

How to Prepare:

1. Preheat your oven to 350 degrees F. Layer a loaf pan with a silicone liner.
2. In a bowl, combine baking powder, coconut flour, and xanthan gum and set it aside.
3. Add cheese to a microwave safe bowl and melt it for 30 seconds in the microwave.
4. Stir in eggs and flour mixture then mix well to form a smooth dough.
5. Spread this dough in a greased loaf pan.
6. Whisk sesame seeds with salt, dried onion, melted butter, and poppyseeds in a shallow dish.
7. Brush the poppyseed mixture over the bread.
8. Bake it for 20 minutes until golden brown.
9. Serve fresh.

Prep Time: 10 minutes
Cooking Time: 20 minutes
Total Time: 30 minutes
Servings: 8

Nutritional Values:

- *Calories 251*
- *Total Fat 24.5 g*
- *Saturated Fat 14.7 g*
- *Cholesterol 165 mg*
- *Sodium 142 mg*
- *Total Carbs 4.3 g*
- *Sugar 0.5 g*
- *Fiber 1 g*
- *Protein 5.9 g*

Savory Sage Bread

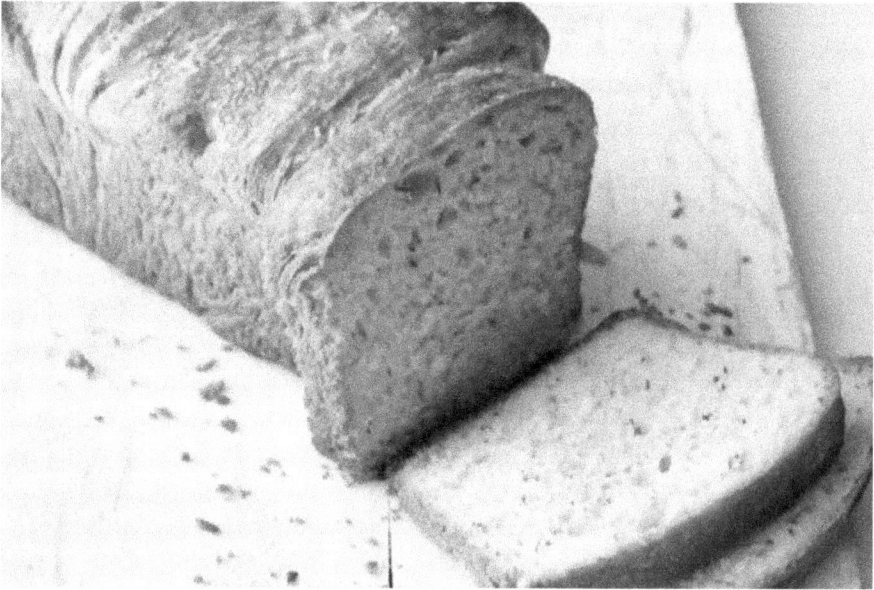

Ingredients:

- 2 ½ cups almond flour
- ¼ cup coconut flour
- ½ cup butter
- 8 oz cream cheese
- 8 whole eggs
- 1 tsp rosemary
- 1 tsp sage
- 2 tbsp parsley
- 1 ½ tsp baking powder

How to Prepare:

1. Beat half cup butter and 8 oz cream cheese in a medium-size bowl with a hand mixer until smooth.

2. Stir in rosemary, parsley, and sage then mix well.
3. Whisk in eggs while beating until mixture is smooth.
4. Add baking powder along with flours and mix well until it forms a thick batter.
5. Grease three small loaf pans and divide the batter into these pans.
6. Place them in the oven and bake the batter for 35 minutes at 350 degrees F.
7. Serve once cooled.

Prep Time: 10 minutes
Cooking Time: 35 minutes
Total Time: 45 minutes
Servings: 12 slices

Nutritional Values:

- *Calories 255*
- *Total Fat 23.4 g*
- *Saturated Fat 11.7 g*
- *Cholesterol 135 mg*
- *Sodium 112 mg*
- *Total Carbs 2.5 g*
- *Sugar 12.5 g*
- *Fiber 1 g*
- *Protein 7.9 g*

Low Carb Flax Bread

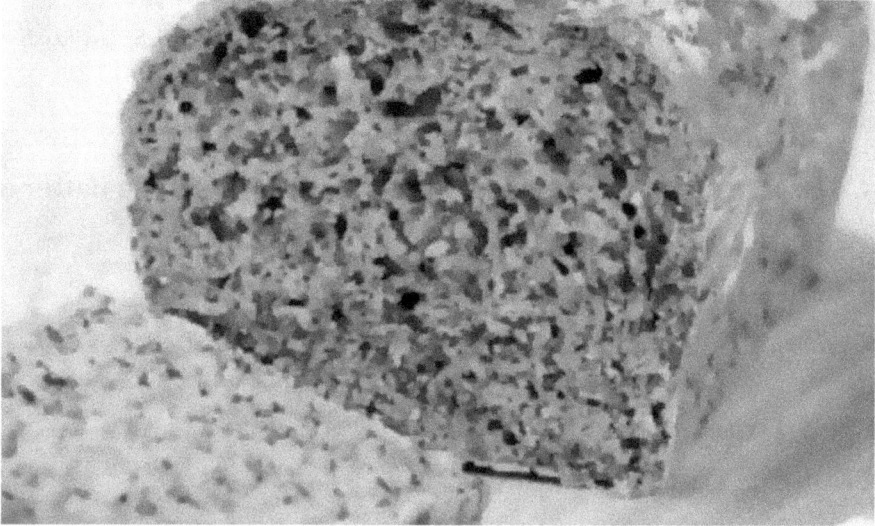

Ingredients:

- ½ cup ground flaxseeds
- ½ cup psyllium husk powder
- 1 tbsp baking powder
- 1 ½ cups soy protein isolate
- ¼ cup granulated stevia
- 2 tsp salt
- 7 large egg whites
- 1 large whole egg
- 3 tbsp butter
- ¾ cup of water

How to Prepare:

1. Preheat your oven to 350 degrees F.

2. Whisk baking powder, ground flaxseed, psyllium husk, stevia, protein, and salt in a bowl.
3. Beat egg with butter, water, and egg whites in a separate bowl.
4. Mix these two mixtures together until smooth.
5. Grease a loaf pan with cooking oil then spread the batter in it.
6. Bake it for 20 minutes until it is done.
7. Enjoy.

Prep Time: 10 minutes
Cooking Time: 20 minutes
Total Time: 30 minutes
Servings: 8 slices

Nutritional Values:
- *Calories 207*
- *Total Fat 19 g*
- *Saturated Fat 14 g*
- *Cholesterol 111 mg*
- *Sodium 122 mg*
- *Total Carbs 7 g*
- *Sugar 1 g*
- *Fiber 3 g*
- *Protein 6 g*

Lemon & Rosemary Shortbread

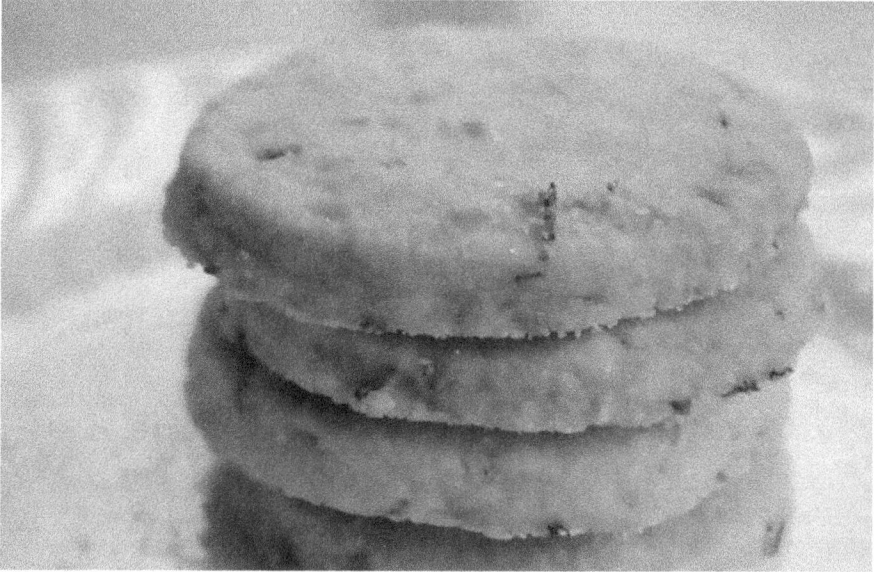

Ingredients:

- 6 tbsp butter
- 2 cups almond flour
- 1/3 cup granulated Swerve
- 1 tbsp freshly grated lemon zest
- 4 tsp fresh squeezed lemon juice
- 1 tsp vanilla extract
- 2 tsp rosemary
- ½ tsp baking soda
- ½ tsp baking powder

How to Prepare:

1. Mix 2 cups of the flour with baking soda and baking powder in a large bowl.
2. Stir in Swerve and mix well then add the lemon zest and lemon juice.
3. Add butter and vanilla to a bowl and heat it in the microwave for 30 seconds on high.
4. Mix well then pour it into the flour mixture along with rosemary.
5. Whisk well until smooth then knead it into a long log.
6. Wrap the dough in plastic wrap. Refrigerate for 30 minutes.
7. Meanwhile, let your oven preheat at 350 degrees F.
8. Remove the wrap and slice the dough log into ½-inch thick slices.
9. Place the slices on a cookie sheet greased with butter.
10. Arrange the dough slices on the baking sheet then bake them for 15 minutes.
11. Let them cool for 10 minutes and serve.

Prep Time: 5 minutes

Cooking Time: 15 minutes

Total Time: 20 minutes

Servings: 10 slices

Nutritional Values:

- *Calories 267*
- *Total Fat 24.5 g*
- *Saturated Fat 17.4 g*
- *Cholesterol 153 mg*
- *Sodium 217 mg*
- *Total Carbs 8.4 g*
- *Sugar 2.3 g*
- *Fiber 1.3 g*
- *Protein 3.1 g*

Spiced Focaccia Bread

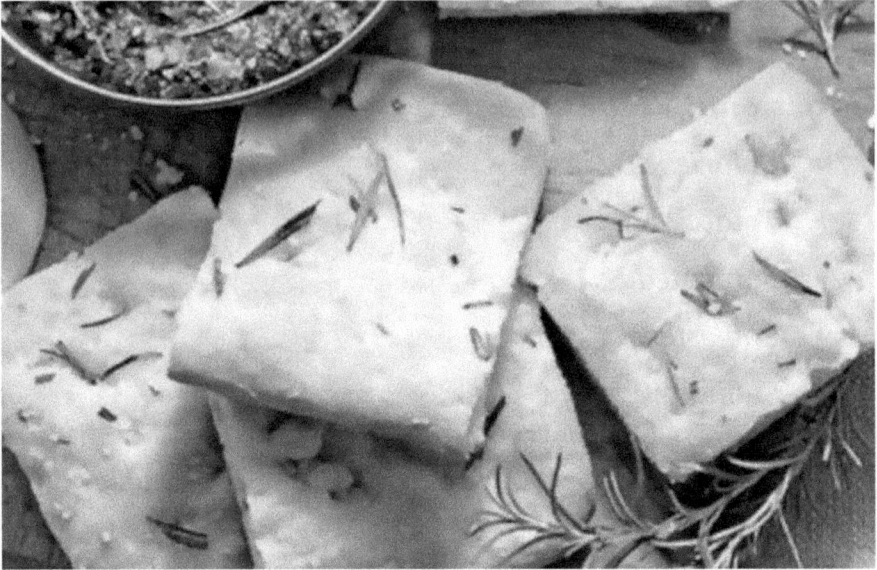

Ingredients:
- 1 cup almond flour
- 1 cup flaxseed meal
- 7 large eggs
- ¼ cup olive oil
- 1 ½ tbsp baking powder
- 2 tsp minced garlic
- 1 tsp salt
- 1 tsp rosemary
- 1 tsp red chili flakes

How to Prepare:
1. Preheat your oven to 350 degrees F.

2. Whisk almond flour with flaxseed meal, spices, and baking powder in a bowl.
3. Stir in garlic, eggs, and olive oil and beat this mixture well until smooth.
4. Grease a 9x9-inch baking pan with cooking spray.
5. Pour the prepared batter in the baking pan then bake for 25 minutes.
6. Allow to cool for 10 minutes then slice.
7. Serve.

Prep Time: 10 minutes
Cooking Time: 25 minutes
Total Time: 35 minutes
Servings: 9 slices

Nutritional Values:

- *Calories 245*
- *Total Fat 19.9 g*
- *Saturated Fat 4.8 g*
- *Cholesterol 32 mg*
- *Sodium 597 mg*
- *Total Carbs 3.4 g*
- *Sugar 1.9 g*
- *Fiber 0.6 g*
- *Protein 10.29 g*

Keto Breadsticks

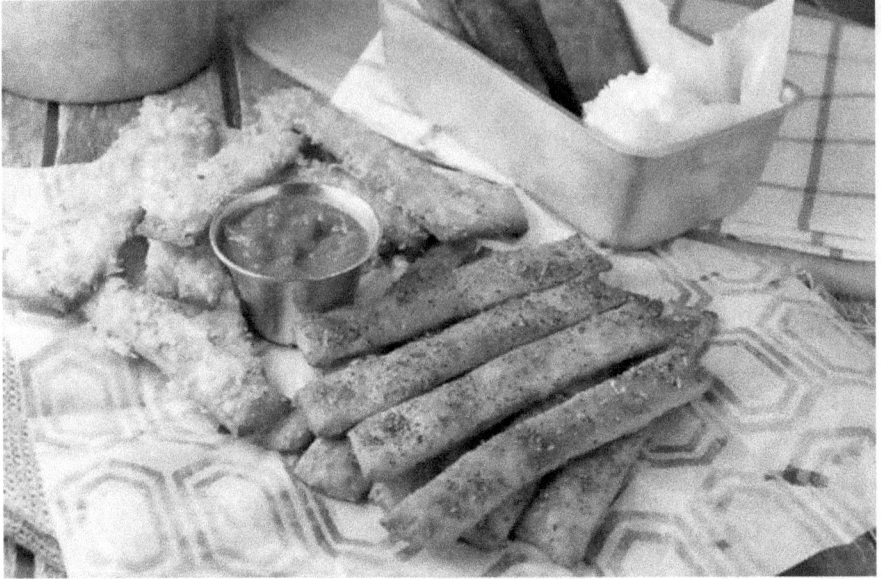

Ingredients:

Bread Stick Base

- 2 cups mozzarella cheese, shredded
- ¾ cup almond flour
- 1 tbsp psyllium husk powder
- 3 tbsp cream cheese
- 1 large egg
- 1 tsp baking powder

Italian Spice Mix

- 2 tbsp Italian seasoning
- 1 tsp salt

- 1 tsp pepper

Extra Cheese Topping
- 1 tsp garlic powder
- 1 tsp onion powder
- 3 oz cheddar cheese
- ¼ cup parmesan cheese

How to prepare:
1. Preheat your oven to 400 degrees F.
2. Whisk egg with cream cheese in a bowl and set it aside.
3. Mix almond flour, baking powder, and psyllium husk in a separate bowl.
4. Heat mozzarella cheese in a large bowl in the microwave for 20 seconds.
5. Mix well then stir in cream cheese, egg, and dry mixture.
6. Continue mixing then knead this dough on your work surface.
7. Spread this dough into a flat thick sheet then place it on a baking sheet.
8. Mix everything for the Italian spice mix and sprinkle it over the dough.

9. Mix everything for the cheese topping and spread that over the dough.

10. Bake the dough for 15 minutes until crispy.

11. Slice into long sticks.

12. Serve with a cream cheese dip or your favourite spread.

13. Enjoy.

Prep Time: 5 minutes

Cooking Time: 15 minutes

Total Time: 20 minutes

Servings: 6 breadsticks

Nutritional Values:

- *Calories 216*
- *Total Fat 20.9 g*
- *Saturated Fat 8.1 g*
- *Cholesterol 241 mg*
- *Total Carbs 8.3 g*
- *Sugar 1.8 g*
- *Fiber 3.8 g*
- *Sodium 8 mg*
- *Protein 6.4 g*

Keto Cream Cheese Bread

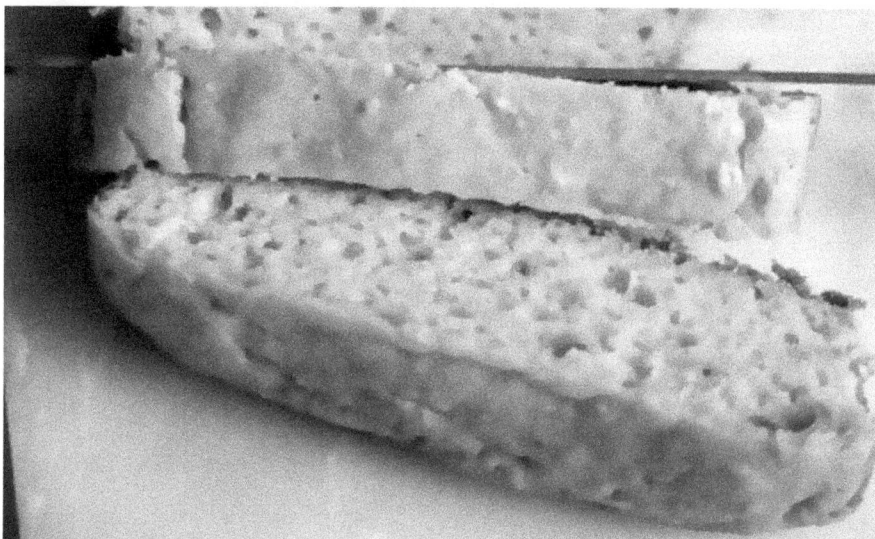

Ingredients:

- 8 large eggs
- 8 oz full-fat cream cheese
- ½ cup unsalted butter
- 1 ½ cups coconut flour
- ½ cup full-fat sour cream
- 4 tsp baking powder
- 1 tsp sea salt
- 1 tbsp Swerve
- 2 tbsp sesame seeds

How to Prepare:

1. Preheat your oven to 350 degrees F.
2. Grease a 10-inch loaf pan with butter liberally.

3. Whisk baking powder, sweetener, salt, and coconut flour together in a medium-size bowl.
4. Beat cream cheese with butter in a bowl until fluffy using a hand mixer.
5. Add eggs one by one while beating the mixture.
6. Add flour mixture and combine until smooth.
7. Fold in the sour cream and mix well until incorporated.
8. Spread this dough into the prepared pan.
9. Bake it for 30 minutes until golden brown.
10. Enjoy.

Prep Time: 5 minutes
Cooking Time: 30 minutes
Total Time: 35 minutes
Servings: 6 slices

Nutritional Values:
- *Calories 282*
- *Total Fat 25.1 g*
- *Saturated Fat 8.8 g*
- *Cholesterol 100 mg*
- *Sodium 117 mg*
- *Total Carbs 9.4 g*
- *Sugar 0.7 g*
- *Fiber 3.2 g*
- *Protein 8 g*

Jalapeno Cornbread Loaves

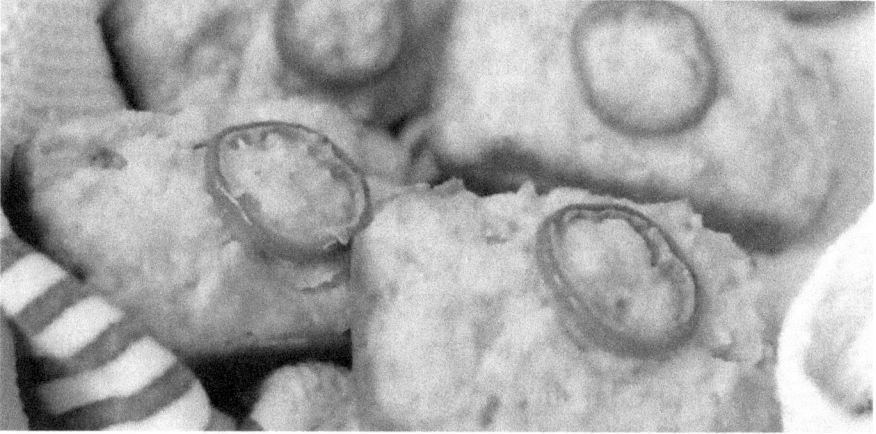

Ingredients:

Dry Ingredients
- 1 ½ cups almond flour
- ½ cup golden flaxseed meal
- 2 tsp baking powder
- 1 tsp salt

Wet Ingredients
- ½ cup sour cream, full fat
- 4 tbsp butter, melted
- 4 large eggs
- 10 drops liquid stevia
- 1 tsp Amoretti sweet corn extract

Add-Ins
- ½ cup sharp cheddar cheese, grated
- 2 fresh jalapenos, seeded and ribs removed
- Sliced jalapenos, for topping

How to Prepare:

1. Preheat your oven to 375 degrees F.
2. Grease a mini loaf pan with cooking oil or butter.
3. Mix almond flour, salt, baking powder, and flaxseed meal in a bowl.
4. Whisk wet ingredients in a separate bowl then stir in the dry mixture.
5. After mixing it well, fold in the chopped pepper and cheddar cheese.
6. Spread this batter evenly in the loaf pan and place additional sliced pepper rings on top.
7. Bake the loaf for 22 minutes until golden brown.
8. Slice and serve.

Prep Time: 5 minutes
Cooking Time: 22 minutes
Total Time: 27 minutes
Servings: 8 slices

Nutritional Values:

- *Calories 301*
- *Total Fat 26.3 g*
- *Saturated Fat 14.8 g*
- *Cholesterol 322 mg*
- *Sodium 597 mg*
- *Total Carbs 2.6 g*
- *Fiber 0.6 g*
- *Sugar 1.9 g*
- *Protein 12 g*

Morning Hamburger Loaves

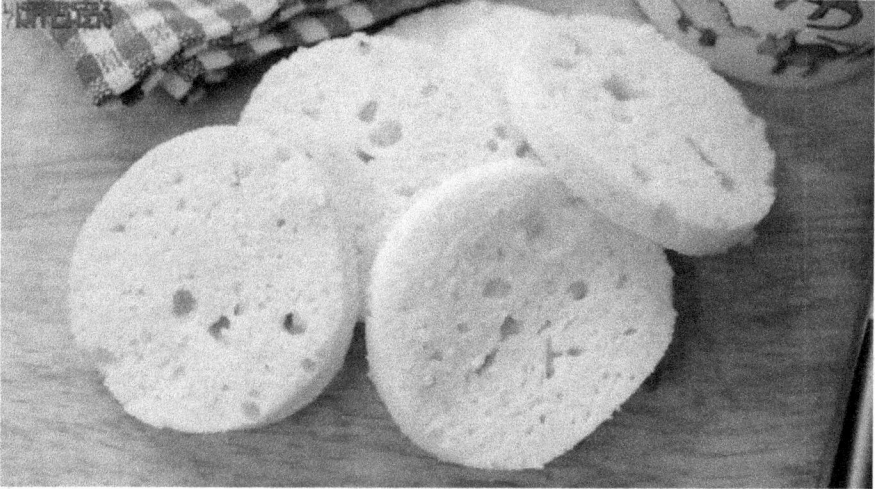

Ingredients:

- 1 large egg
- 1 tbsp almond flour
- 1 tbsp psyllium husk powder
- ¼ tsp baking powder
- ¼ tsp cream of tartar
- 1 tbsp chicken broth
- 1 tbsp melted butter

How to Prepare:

1. Crack an egg in a wide microwave-safe mug.
2. Pour melted butter over the egg and let it sit for 1 minute.

3. Stir in almond flour, baking powder, chicken broth, cream of tartar, and husk powder.

4. Mix well to form a smooth batter then place the mug in the microwave.

5. Bake it for 75 seconds in the microwave on High.

6. Slice and serve.

Prep Time: 5 minutes
Cooking Time: 1.5 minutes
Total Time: 6.5 minutes
Servings: 1

Nutritional Values:

- *Calories 248*
- *Total Fat 19.3 g*
- *Saturated Fat 4.8 g*
- *Cholesterol 32 mg*
- *Sodium 597 mg*
- *Total Carbs 3.1 g*
- *Fiber 0.6 g*
- *Sugar 1.9 g*
- *Protein 7.9 g*

Cheesy Keto Garlic Bread

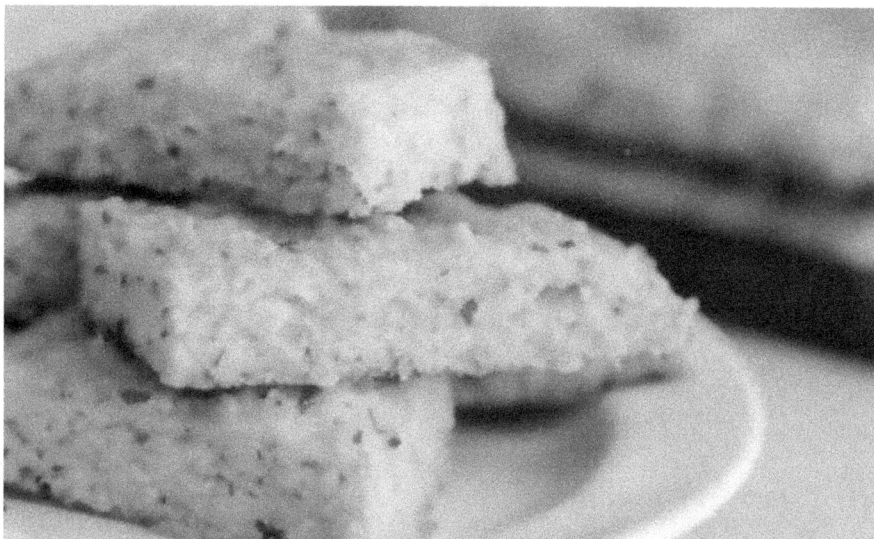

Ingredients:

- 1¾ cups grated cheese mozzarella
- ¾ cups almond flour
- 2 tbsp cream cheese, full fat
- 1 tsp baking powder
- Pinch salt, to taste
- 1 medium egg

Glaze:

- 1 tbsp garlic, crushed
- 1 tbsp parsley, fresh or dried
- 2 tbsp butter, melted

How to Prepare:

1. Add everything except the egg to a microwave-safe bowl.

2. Heat this mixture for 1 minute in the microwave on High.
3. Stir well then heat again for 30 seconds in the microwave.
4. Whisk in egg and stir well to form the dough.
5. Spread this dough in a greased loaf pan and set aside.
6. Prepare the glaze by mixing butter with garlic.
7. Brush this mixture liberally over the bread.
8. Bake for 15 minutes at 425 degrees F until golden.
9. Enjoy.

Prep Time: 5 minutes
Cooking Time: 15 minutes
Total Time: 20 minutes
Servings: 6 slices

Nutritional Values:
- *Calories 158*
- *Total Fat 15.2 g*
- *Saturated Fat 5.2 g*
- *Cholesterol 269 mg*
- *Sodium 178 mg*
- *Total Carbs 7.4 g*
- *Sugar 1.1 g*
- *Fiber 3.5 g*
- *Protein 5.5 g*

Apple Cider Bread

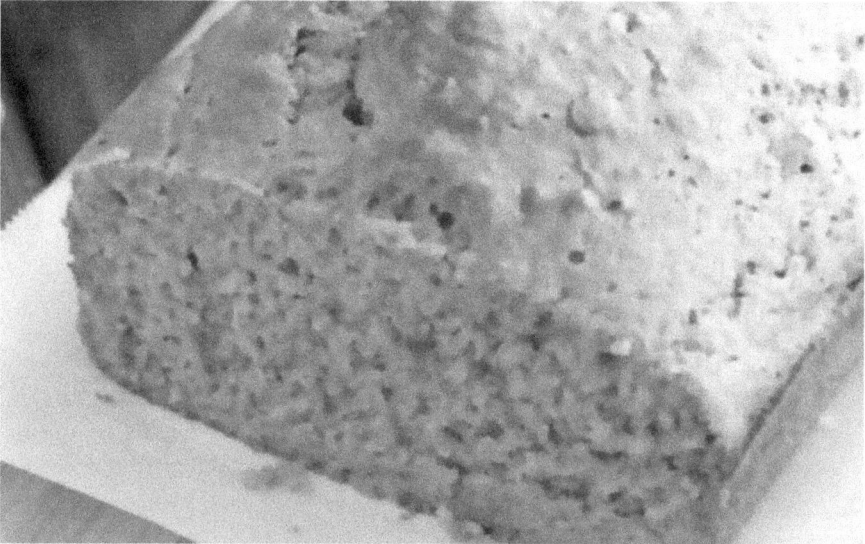

Ingredients:
- 1 egg
- 1/3 cup sour cream
- 1 tbsp + 2 tsp apple cider vinegar
- 2 tbsp water
- 1 cup almond flour
- 5 tbsp golden flaxseed meal
- 3 tbsp coconut flour
- 1/3 cup whey protein isolate
- 3 ½ tsp baking powder
- 1 tsp xanthan gum
- ½ tsp kosher salt
- 8 tbsp butter, melted

How to Prepare:
1. Preheat your oven to 350 degrees F.

2. Layer a baking tray with wax paper and set it aside.
3. Beat eggs with apple cider vinegar, water, and sour cream in a medium bowl.
4. Grind flaxseed meal with almond flour, whey protein, coconut flour, salt, baking powder, and xanthan gum in a food processor.
5. Add butter and egg mixture and blend again until smooth.
6. Spread the batter in the baking tray.
7. Brush the top with melted butter then bake for 20 minutes.
8. Let them cool for 10 minutes.
9. Slice and serve.

Prep Time: 10 minutes
Cooking Time: 20 minutes
Total Time: 30 minutes
Servings: 6

Nutritional Values:
- *Calories 214*
- *Total Fat 19 g*
- *Saturated Fat 5.8 g*
- *Cholesterol 15 mg*
- *Sodium 123 mg*
- *Total Carbs 6.5 g*
- *Sugar 1.9 g*
- *Fiber 2.1 g*
- *Protein 6.5 g*

Turmeric Cauliflower Bread

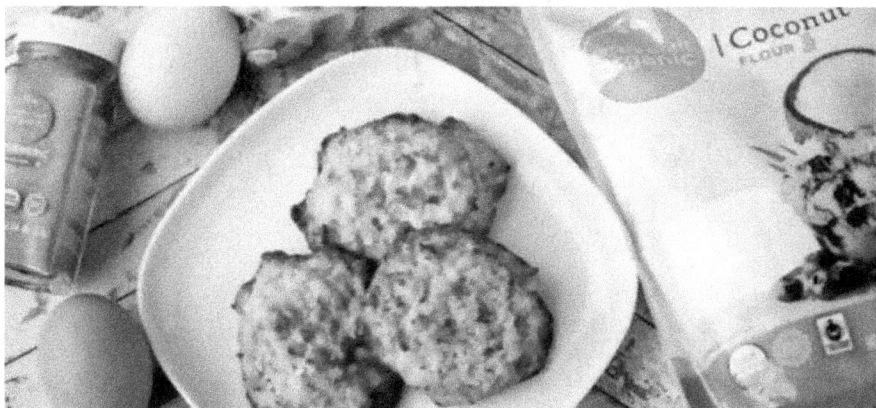

Ingredients:

- 2 cups cauliflower rice
- 2 eggs
- 2 tbsp coconut flour
- ¼ tsp ground turmeric
- Pinch each of salt and pepper

How to Prepare:

1. Preheat your oven to 400 degrees F. Layer a baking sheet with wax paper.
2. Add a teaspoon of water to the cauliflower rice in a microwave safe bowl.
3. Cook for 3 minutes on High.
4. Transfer the cauliflower rice to a kitchen towel and squeeze out excess water.

5. Mix drained cauliflower rice with coconut flour, eggs, salt, black pepper, and turmeric in a bowl.
6. Make 6 equal-sized rounds out of this mixture and place them in a baking sheet.
7. Bake them for 30 minutes until golden brown.
8. Serve.

Prep Time: 10 minutes
Cooking Time: 30 minutes
Total Time: 40 minutes
Servings: 6

Nutritional Values:

- *Calories 113*
- *Total Fat 8.4 g*
- *Saturated Fat 12.1 g*
- *Cholesterol 27 mg*
- *Sodium 39 mg*
- *Total Carbs 9.2 g*
- *Sugar 3.1 g*
- *Fiber 4.6 g*
- *Protein 8.1 g*

Keto Bagel Loaves

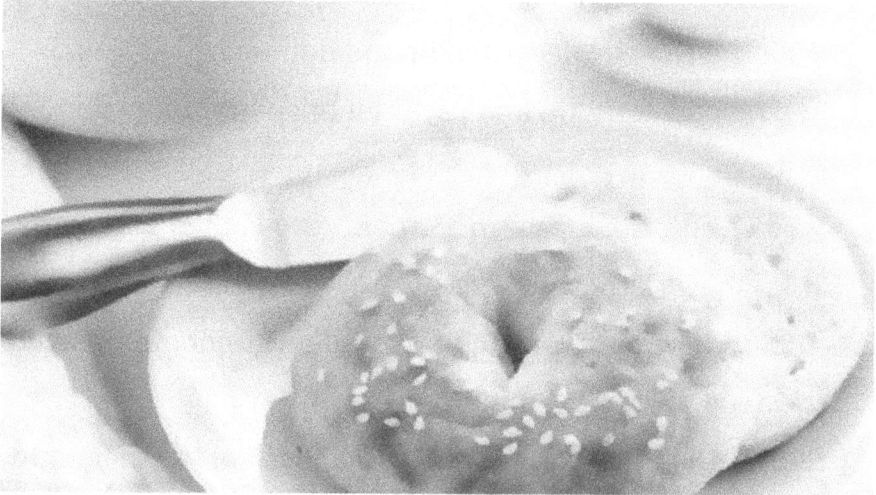

Ingredients:

- 1 cup almond flour
- ¼ cup coconut flour
- 1 tbsp psyllium husk powder
- 1 tsp baking powder
- 1 tsp garlic powder
- Pinch salt
- 2 medium eggs
- 2 tsp white wine vinegar
- 2 ½ tbsp ghee, melted
- 1 tbsp olive oil
- 1 tsp sesame seeds

How to Prepare:

1. Preheat your oven to 320 degrees F.
2. Whisk garlic powder with almond flour, coconut flour, baking powder, salt, and psyllium husk powder in a suitable bowl.
3. Beat eggs with vinegar in a separate bowl then stir in ghee slowly while still whisking.
4. Add dry flour mixture and mix well until smooth then let the dough rest for 3 minutes.
5. Slice the dough into 4 equal pieces then spread them into thick rounds.
6. Place them onto a baking sheet layered with parchment paper.
7. Cut a small hole in the center of each round using a cookie cutter.
8. Sprinkle sesame seeds on top then bake for 25 minutes.
9. Enjoy.

Prep Time: 10 minutes
Cooking Time: 25 minutes
Total Time: 35 minutes
Servings: 4

Nutritional Values:

- *Calories 220*
- *Total Fat 20.1 g*
- *Saturated Fat 7.4 g*
- *Cholesterol 132 mg*
- *Sodium 157 mg*
- *Total Carbs 63 g*
- *Sugar 0.4 g*
- *Fiber 2.4 g*
- *Protein 6.1 g*

Chapter 4 No Carb Keto Cookies

Peanut Butter Cookies

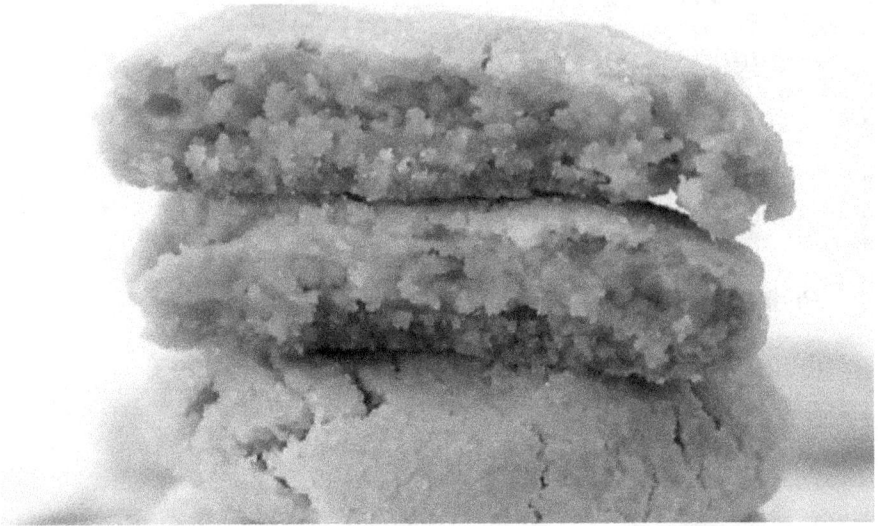

Ingredients:

- ½ cup peanut butter
- ½ cup powdered erythritol
- 1 egg

How to Prepare:

1. Preheat your oven to 350 degrees F.
2. Layer a baking sheet with wax paper and set it aside.

3. Add all the ingredients to a bowl and mix well to prepare the cookie dough.
4. Add 1.5 tablespoons of the dough on the baking sheet scoop by scoop to make the cookies.
5. Bake for 15 minutes until golden brown.
6. Enjoy.

Prep Time: 5 minutes
Cooking Time: 15 minutes
Total Time: 20 minutes
Servings: 4

Nutritional Values:

- *Calories 179*
- *Total Fat 15.7 g*
- *Saturated Fat 8 g*
- *Cholesterol 323mg*
- *Sodium 43 mg*
- *Total Carbs 4.8 g*
- *Sugar 3.6 g*
- *Fiber 0.8 g*
- *Protein 5.6 g*

Mint Creme Oreos

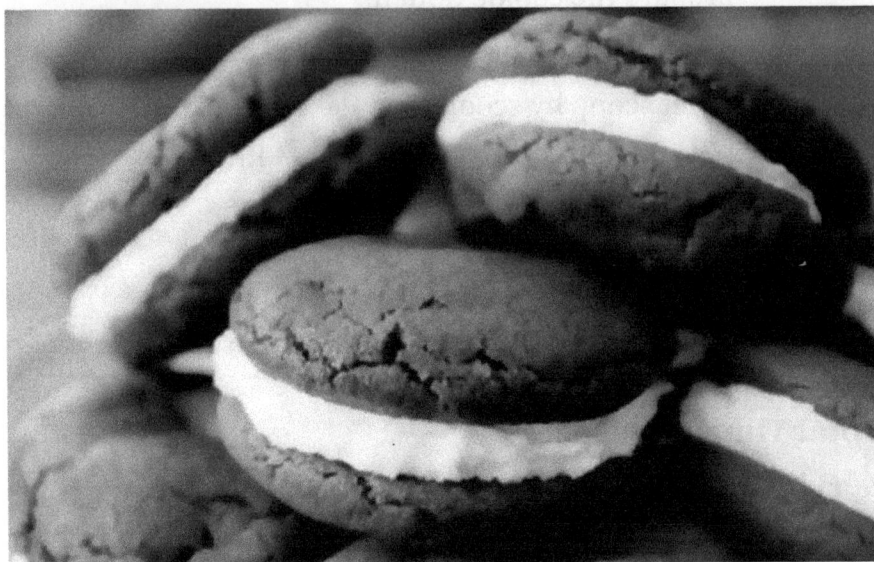

Ingredients:

- 2 ¼ cups almond flour
- 3 tbsp coconut flour
- 4 tbsp cacao powder
- 1 tsp baking powder
- 1 ½ tsp xanthan gum
- ¼ tsp salt
- ½ cup grass-fed butter, unsalted and softened
- 1 egg
- 1 tsp vanilla extract
- 4 oz cream cheese
- 1 cup lakanto monk fruit

- 1 tsp peppermint extract

How to Prepare:

1. Preheat your oven to 350 degrees F.
2. Mix coconut flour with almond flour, xanthan gum, salt, baking powder, and cocoa powder in a medium-sized bowl.
3. Whisk ½ cup monk fruit sweetener with six tablespoons of butter in a bowl until fluffy.
4. Add vanilla extract and egg then beat well and stir in dry ingredients to form the dough.
5. Place this dough in between two sheets of wax paper and roll it into a 1/8-inch thick sheet.
6. Cut cookies with a round cookie cutter then re-roll the remaining dough to cut more cookies.
7. Place these cookies on a cookie sheet lined with parchment paper.
8. Bake these cookies for 12 minutes then allow them to cool.
9. Meanwhile, beat cream cheese with 2 tablespoons butter, ½ cup monk fruit, and peppermint extract in a small bowl.
10. Divide this mixture over half of the cookies.
11. Place the remaining half of the cookies over the cream filling.

12.   Press the two halves together gently.

13.   Enjoy.

Prep Time: 10 minutes

Cooking Time: 12 minutes

Total Time: 22 minutes

Servings: 12

Nutritional Values:

- *Calories 331*
- *Total Fat 12.9 g*
- *Saturated Fat 6.1 g*
- *Cholesterol 10 mg*
- *Sodium 18 mg*
- *Total Carbs 9.1 g*
- *Sugar 2.8 g*
- *Fiber 0.8 g*
- *Protein 4.4 g*

Butter Glazed Cookies

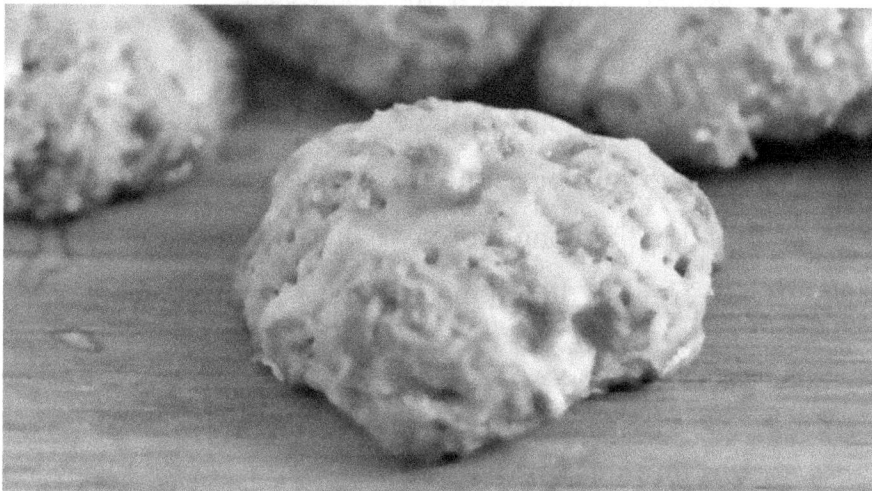

Ingredients:

- 1/3 cup coconut flour
- 2/3 cup almond flour
- ¼ cup granulated erythritol
- 8 drops stevia
- ½ cup butter, softened
- 1 tsp almond or vanilla extract
- ¼ tsp baking powder
- ¼ tsp xanthan gum (optional)

For the Glaze:

- ¼ cup coconut butter
- 8 drops stevia

How to Prepare:

1. Preheat your oven to 356 degrees F.
2. Whisk dry ingredients in one bowl and beat butter with stevia and vanilla extract in another.
3. Add dry mixture and mix well until smooth then divide the dough into two pieces.
4. Place each dough piece in between two sheets of wax paper.
5. Spread them into a thick sheet and refrigerate for 10 minutes.
6. Use a cookies cutter to cut small cookies out of both the dough sheets.
7. Place them on a baking sheet lined with wax paper and bake them for 6 minutes.
8. Meanwhile, prepare the glaze by heating coconut butter with stevia in a bowl in the microwave.
9. Pour this glaze over each cookie and allow it to set.
10. Serve.

Prep Time: 15 minutes
Cooking Time: 6 minutes
Total Time: 21 minutes
Servings: 40 cookies

Nutritional Values:

- *Calories 237*
- *Total Fat 22 g*
- *Saturated Fat 9 g*
- *Cholesterol 35 mg*
- *Sodium 118 mg*
- *Total Carbs 5 g*
- *Sugar 1 g*
- *Fiber 2 g*
- *Protein 5 g*

Keto Thumbprint Cookies

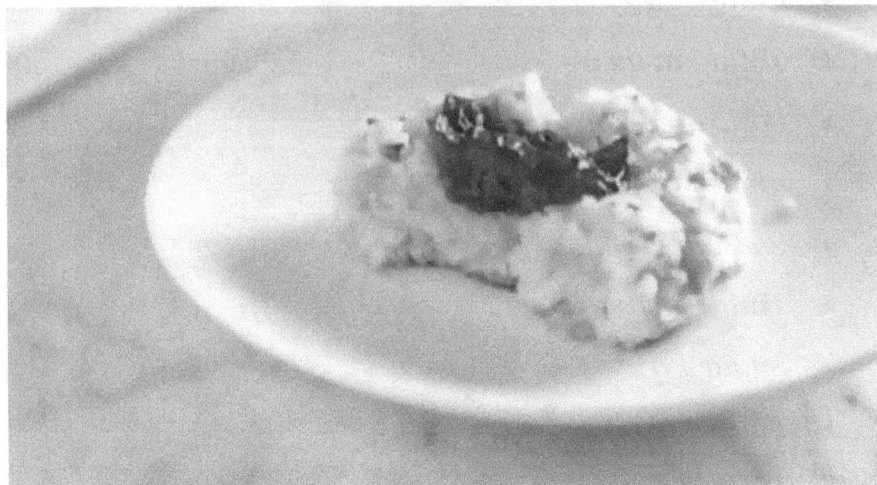

Ingredients:

- 1 large egg, beaten
- ½ cup salted butter, softened
- 2 cups superfine blanched almond flour
- Pinch of kosher salt
- ½ tsp baking powder
- 2/3 cup powdered erythritol sweetener
- 1 tsp vanilla extract
- 1/3 cup finely chopped walnuts
- 5 tbsp sugar-free strawberry preserves

How to Prepare:

1. Preheat your oven to 375 degrees F.
2. Beat egg with almond flour, vanilla, butter, salt, erythritol, baking powder, and vanilla in a medium bowl.

3. Make 1.5-inch balls out of this mixture and flatten them slightly.
4. Top these cookies with the walnuts then place them on a baking sheet lined with wax paper.
5. Bake them for 8 minutes then make small grooves in the center of each cookie.
6. Add a teaspoon of jam into the center of each cookie then bake them for 10 minutes.
7. Let them cool down completely.
8. Serve.

Prep Time: 10 minutes
Cooking Time: 8 minutes
Total Time: 18 minutes
Servings: 8

Nutritional Values:
- *Calories 190*
- *Total Fat 17.5 g*
- *Saturated Fat 7.1 g*
- *Cholesterol 20 mg*
- *Sodium 28 mg*
- *Total Carbs 5.5 g*
- *Sugar 2.8 g*
- *Fiber 3.8 g*
- *Protein 3 g*

Pecan Shortbread Cookies

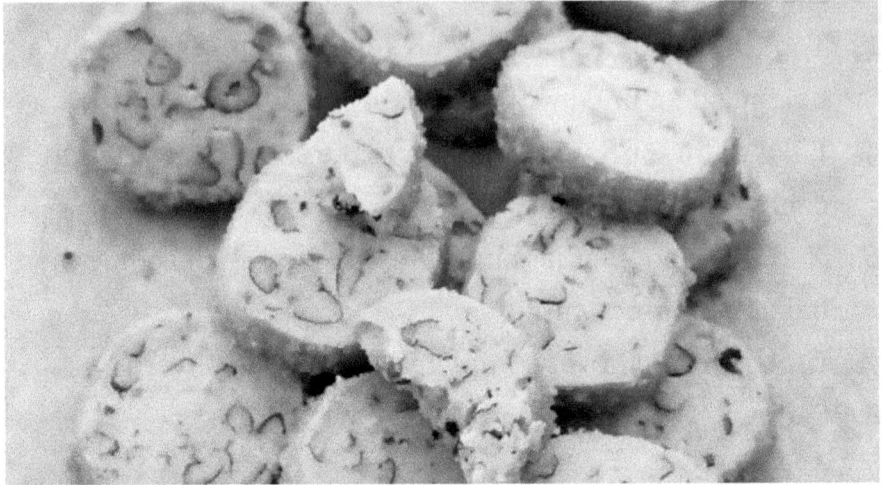

Ingredients:

- ¾ cup almond flour
- ¼ cup coconut flour
- 1 large egg
- 4 tbsp butter, melted
- ½ cup erythritol
- 1 tsp vanilla extract
- ½ tsp baking powder
- ¼ tsp xanthan gum
- 1/3 cup raw pecans, crushed

How to Prepare:

1. Add all dry ingredients to a bowl then mix well with a fork.

2. Whisk melted butter and vanilla extract in a separate bowl then stir in half of the dry mixture.

3. Add egg and mix well until combined. Now, stir in the remaining dry mixture.

4. Mix this well until fully incorporated.

5. Add pecans to the cookie dough and mix well.

6. Place the dough on wax paper and form it into a rectangular log with your hands.

7. Cover it with more wax paper and freeze for 30 minutes.

8. Meanwhile, preheat your oven for 5 minutes at 350 degrees F.

9. Layer a cookie sheet with wax paper and set it aside.

10. Slice the dough log into ¼-inch thick slices.

11. Place the slices on the cookie sheet and bake them for 15 minutes.

12. Allow them to cool then serve.

Prep Time: 5 minutes
Cooking Time: 15 minutes
Total Time: 20 minutes
Servings: 6

Nutritional Values:

- *Calories 121*
- *Total Fat 12.9 g*
- *Saturated Fat 5.1 g*
- *Cholesterol 17 mg*
- *Sodium 28 mg*
- *Total Carbs 8.1 g*
- *Sugar 1.8 g*
- *Fiber 0.4 g*
- *Protein 5.4 g*

Pistachio Cookies

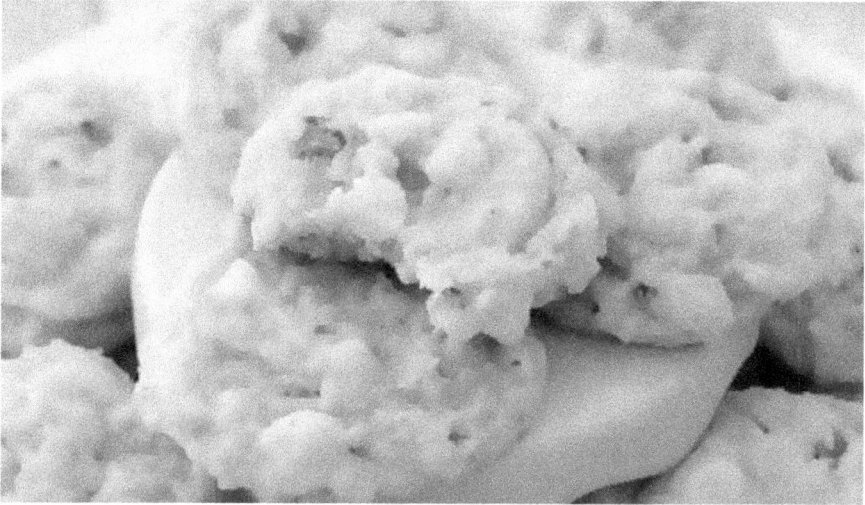

Ingredients:

- ¾ cup (4 oz) shelled pistachio nuts
- 2 tsp + 1 cup stevia granulated sweetener
- 1 2/3 cup almond meal or almond flour
- 2 eggs, beaten well

How to Prepare:

1. Add pistachio and stevia to a food processor and pulse until finely ground.
2. Toss pistachio mixture with almond meal or flour in a bowl.
3. Add eggs and whisk well until combined.
4. Refrigerate this mixture for 8 hours or overnight.
5. Let your oven preheat at 325 degrees F.

6. Layer a cookie sheet with wax paper then use a scoop or spoon to add the cookie dough to the sheet scoop by scoop.
7. Bake them for 25 minutes until lightly brown.
8. Allow them to cool then serve.

Prep Time: 10 minutes

Cooking Time: 25 minutes

Total Time: 35 minutes

Servings: 8

Nutritional Values:

- *Calories 174*
- *Total Fat 12.3 g*
- *Saturated Fat 4.8 g*
- *Cholesterol 32 mg*
- *Sodium 597 mg*
- *Total Carbs 4.5 g*
- *Fiber 0.6 g*
- *Sugar 1.9 g*
- *Protein 12 g*

Chocolate Dipped Cookies

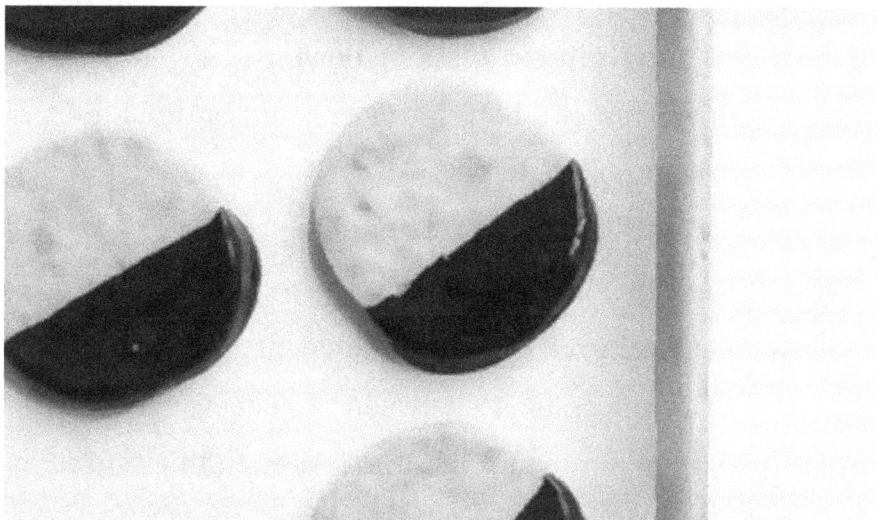

Ingredients:

- 1 ½ cups almond flour
- ¼ cup almond butter
- 2 tbsp powdered erythritol
- 1 large egg
- 1 tsp vanilla powder
- 1 tbsp virgin coconut oil
- 1 tbsp coconut butter
- 1 tsp baking powder
- Pinch of salt
- 3.2 oz 90% dark chocolate

How to Prepare:

1. Whisk almond flour, vanilla, salt, baking powder, and erythritol in a mixing bowl.
2. Stir in almond butter, egg, coconut butter, and coconut oil.
3. Mix well to form a dough then place it in a sandwich bag. Refrigerate for 30 minutes.
4. Let your oven preheat at 285 degrees F.
5. Place the dough in between two sheets of parchment then roll it into a ½-inch thick sheet.
6. Use a 2.5-inch diameter cookie cutter to cut the cookies out of this dough.
7. Reroll the remaining dough then place it on a greased baking sheet.
8. Bake the cookies for 30 minutes until golden brown.
9. Place them on a wire rack to cool down.
10. Melt chocolate in a bowl by heating in a microwave and stir well.
11. Dip half of each cooled cookie in the chocolate melt and allow it to set on wax paper.
12. Refrigerate the dipped cookies for 15 minutes.
13. Serve.

Prep Time: 10 minutes

Cooking Time: 30 minutes

Total Time: 40 minutes

Servings: 8

Nutritional Values:

- *Calories 236*
- *Total Fat 13.5 g*
- *Saturated Fat 4.2 g*
- *Cholesterol 541 mg*
- *Sodium 21 mg*
- *Total Carbs 7.6 g*
- *Sugar 1.4 g*
- *Fiber 3.8 g*
- *Protein 4.3 g*

Shortbread Cookies

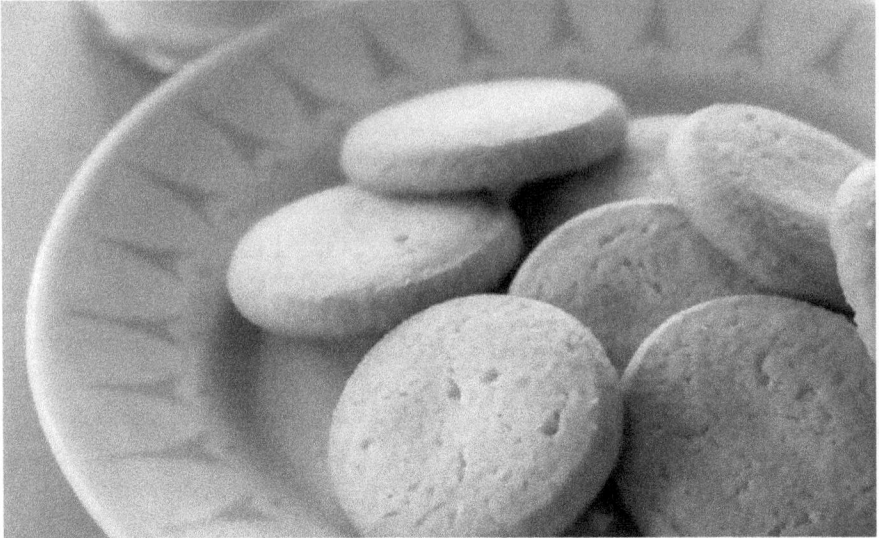

Ingredients:

- 1 ½ cups almond flour
- ½ tsp xanthan gum
- ¼ tsp kosher salt
- 6 tbsp grass-fed butter, room temperature
- 6 tbsp powdered erythritol
- ½ tsp vanilla extract

How to Prepare:

1. Spread almond flour in a dry skillet and place it over medium heat.

2. Stir cook for 3 minutes or more until golden brown then remove it from the heat.

3. Add salt and xanthan gum to the flour and mix well.

4. Beat butter with an electric mixer for 3 minutes and add sweetener.

5. Continue beating then add vanilla extract. Beat until combined.

6. Add almond flour mixture and whisk well until it forms a smooth dough.

7. Wrap the dough in a plastic wrap then refrigerate for 1 hour.

8. Let your oven preheat at 350 degrees F and grease a baking tray with cooking oil.

9. Place the cookie dough between two parchment sheets and roll it into a ¼-inch thick sheet.

10. Cut out cookies using any shape cookie cutter.

11. Arrange all the cookies on a baking sheet and freeze for 15 minutes.

12. Bake them for 13 minutes until golden brown.

13. Serve.

Prep Time: 10 minutes

Cooking Time: 13 minutes

Total Time: 23 minutes

Servings: 6

Nutritional Values:

- *Calories 167*
- *Total Fat 5.1 g*
- *Saturated Fat 1.1 g*
- *Cholesterol 121 mg*
- *Sodium 48 mg*
- *Total Carbs 8.9 g*
- *Sugar 3.8 g*
- *Fiber 2.1 g*
- *Protein 6.3 g*

Pumpkin Cheesecake Cookies

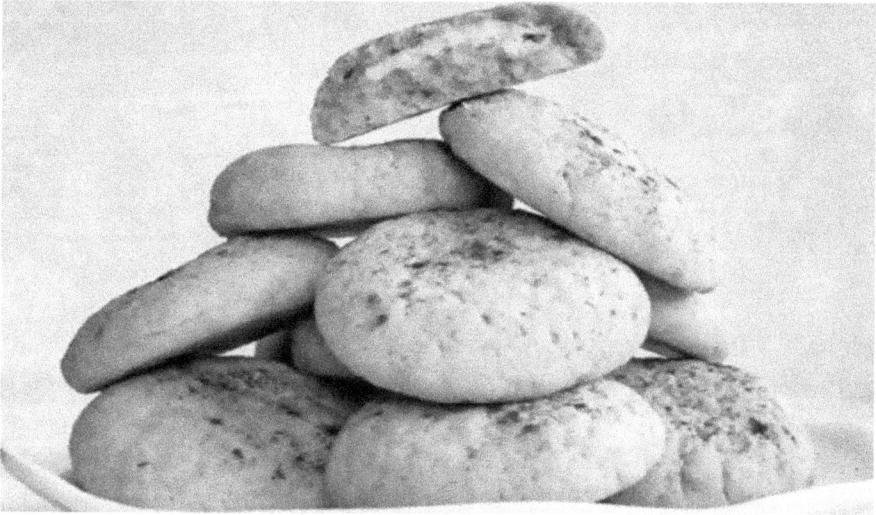

Ingredients:

For the Pumpkin Cookie

- 6 tbsp butter, softened
- 2 cups almond flour
- 1/3 cup solid pack pumpkin puree
- 1 large egg
- ¾ cup granulated erythritol sweetener
- ½ tsp baking powder
- 1 tsp ground cinnamon
- ¼ tsp ground nutmeg
- 1/8 tsp ground allspice
- Pinch of salt

For the Cheesecake Filling

- 4 oz cream cheese
- ½ tsp vanilla
- 1 large egg
- 2 tbsp granulated erythritol sweetener

How to Prepare:

1. Preheat your oven at 350 degrees F.
2. Add all the cookie dough ingredients to a suitable bowl and form a smooth dough.
3. Add the dough to a cookie sheet lined with wax paper scoop by scoop.
4. Flatten the scoops of dough with a spoon and make a dent in the center of each cookie.
5. Whisk cream cheese with vanilla, egg, and sweetener in a mixer.
6. Divide this mixture into the center of each cookie.
7. Bake them for 20 minutes until golden brown.
8. Allow them to cool for 10 minutes.
9. Enjoy.

Prep Time: 10 minutes

Cooking Time: 20 minutes

Total Time: 30 minutes

Servings: 12

Nutritional Values:

- Calories 175
- Total Fat 16 g
- Saturated Fat 2.1 g
- Cholesterol 124 mg
- Sodium 8 mg
- Total Carbs 2.8 g
- Sugar 1.8 g
- Fiber 0.4 g
- *Protein 9 g*

Keto Chocolate Chip Cookies

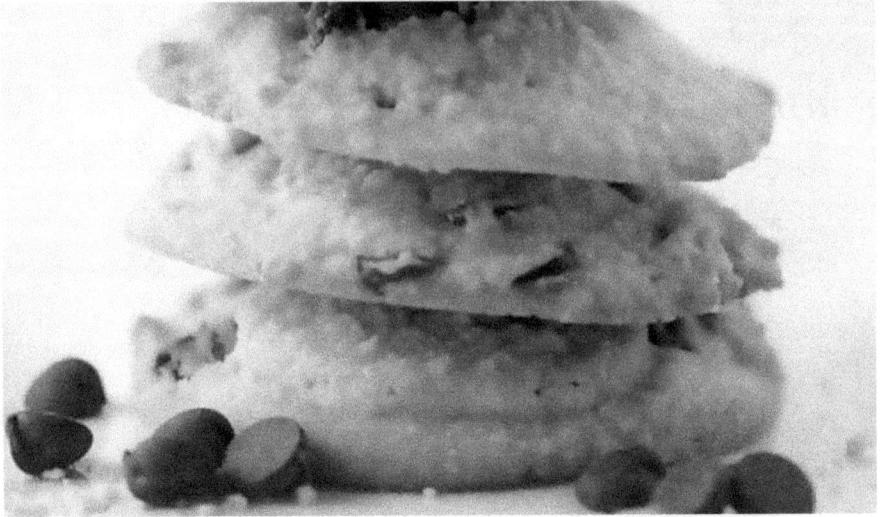

Ingredients:

- 1 cup sunflower seed butter
- 2 eggs
- ¼ cup coconut flour
- 1 tsp vanilla extract
- 1 cup granulated erythritol sweetener
- ¼ cup unsweetened shredded coconut
- 1 tbsp konjac flour
- ¼ tsp kosher salt
- 2 oz coarsely chopped Lindt 90% dark chocolate

How to Prepare:

1. Preheat your oven to 350 degrees F.

2. Mix sunflower seed butter with vanilla, coconut flour, eggs, sweetener, shredded coconut, salt, and konjac flour in a suitably sized bowl.
3. Mix well then fold in chopped chocolate.
4. Make 15 balls out of this mixture then place them on a baking sheet lined with wax paper.
5. Gently press the balls to flatten them into cookies.
6. Bake these cookies for 16 minutes until golden brown.
7. Allow them to cool then garnish with salt flakes.
8. Enjoy.

Prep Time: 10 minutes
Cooking Time: 16 minutes
Total Time: 26 minutes
Servings: 8

Nutritional Values:
- *Calories 285*
- *Total Fat 17.3 g*
- *Saturated Fat 4.5 g*
- *Cholesterol 175 mg*
- *Sodium 165 mg*
- *Total Carbs 3.5 g*
- *Sugar 0.4 g*
- *Fiber 0.9 g*
- *Protein 7.2 g*

Stuffed Oreo Cookies

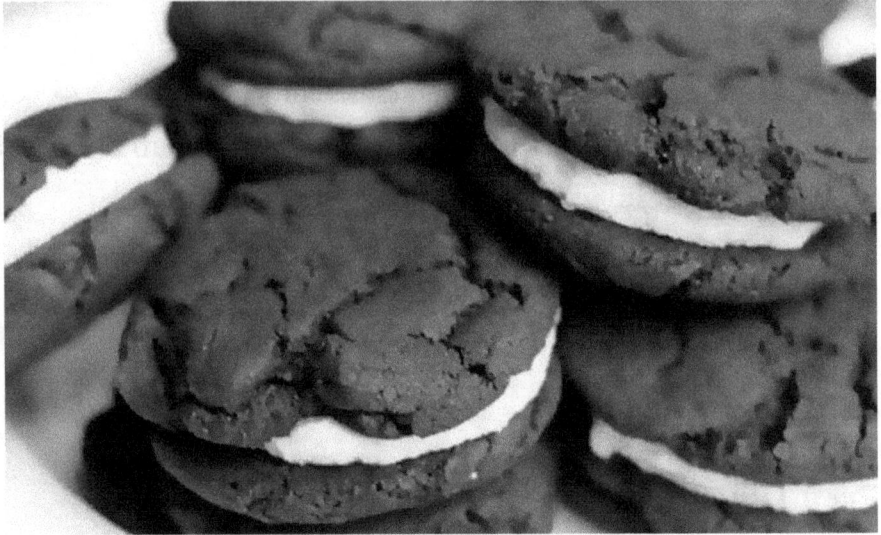

Ingredients:

- 1 1/3 cup almond flour
- 6 tbsp cocoa powder
- 2 tbsp black cocoa powder
- ¾ tsp kosher salt
- ½ tsp xanthan gum
- ½ tsp baking soda
- ¼ tsp espresso powder
- 5 ½ tbsp butter
- 8 tbsp erythritol
- 1 egg

For Vanilla Cream Filling

- 4 tbsp grass-fed butter

- 1 tbsp coconut oil
- 1 ½ tsp vanilla extract
- Pinch kosher salt
- ½ - 1 cup Swerve confectioner sugar substitute

How to Prepare:

1. Whisk almond flour, salt, both cocoa powders, xanthan gum, baking soda, and espresso powder in a suitable bowl.
2. Beat butter well in a large bowl with a hand mixer for 2 minutes.
3. Whisk in sweetener and continue beating for 5 minutes then add the egg.
4. Beat well then add the flour mixture. Mix well until fully incorporated.
5. Wrap the cookie dough with plastic wrap and refrigerate for 1 hour.
6. Meanwhile, preheat your oven to 350 degrees F and layer a baking sheet with wax paper.
7. Place the dough in between two sheets of parchment paper.
8. Roll the dough out into a 1/8-inch thick sheet.
9. Cut 1 ¾ inch round cookies out of this sheet and reroll the dough to cut more cookies.
10. Spread these cookies on the baking sheet and freeze for 15 minutes.
11. Bake these cookies for 12 minutes then allow them to cool on a wire rack.

12. Beat butter with coconut oil in a bowl with an electric mixer.
13. Stir in vanilla extract, powdered sweetener to taste, and a pinch of salt.
14. Mix well then transfer it to a piping bag.
15. Place half of the cookies on a cookie sheet and top them with the cream filling.
16. Place the remaining half of the cookies over the filling to cover it.
17. Refrigerate for 15 minutes then serve.

Prep Time: 5 minutes
Cooking Time: 12 minutes
Total Time: 17 minutes
Servings: 8

Nutritional Values:
- *Calories 215*
- *Total Fat 20 g*
- *Saturated Fat 7 g*
- *Cholesterol 38 mg*
- *Sodium 12 mg*
- *Total Carbs 8 g*
- *Sugar 1 g*
- *Fiber 6 g*
- *Protein 5 g*

Snickerdoodles

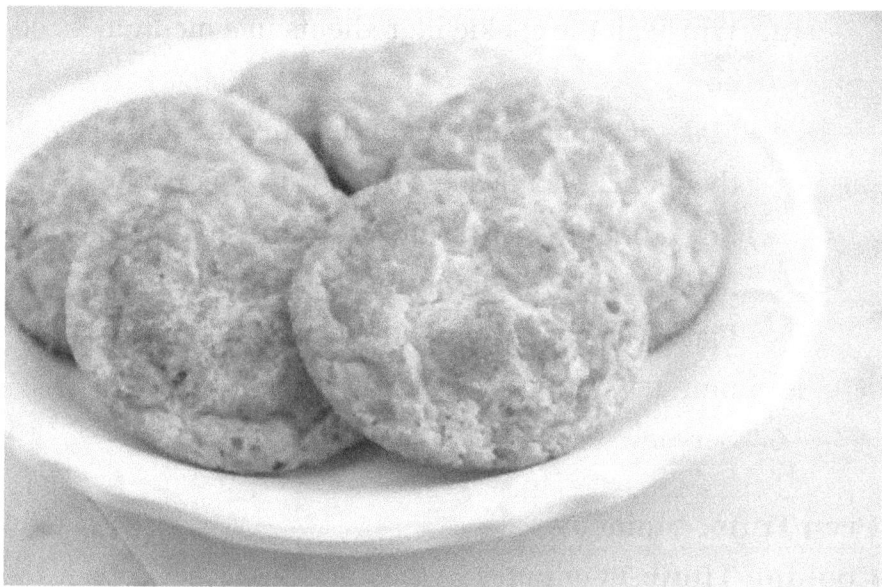

Ingredients:

For the Cookies:

- 2 cups superfine almond flour
- ½ cup salted butter, softened
- Pinch of kosher salt
- ¾ cup erythritol granulated sweetener
- ½ tsp baking soda

For the Coating:

- 2 tbsp erythritol granulated sweetener
- 1 tsp ground cinnamon

How to Prepare:

1. Preheat your oven to 350 degrees F.
2. Whisk all the cookie ingredients in a medium-sized bowl.
3. Make 16 small balls out of this mixture and place them on a baking sheet lined with wax paper.
4. Mix cinnamon with sweetener in a shallow dish and sprinkle this mixture over the balls.
5. Flatten the balls lightly then bake them for 15 minutes.
6. Serve.

Prep Time: 5 minutes
Cooking Time: 15 minutes
Total Time: 20 minutes
Servings: 12

Nutritional Values:

- *Calories 198*
- *Total Fat 19.2 g*
- *Saturated Fat 11.5 g*
- *Cholesterol 123 mg*
- *Sodium 142 mg*
- *Total Carbs 4.5 g*
- *Sugar 3.3 g*
- *Fiber 0.3 g*
- *Protein 3.4 g*

Fudgy Brownie Cookies

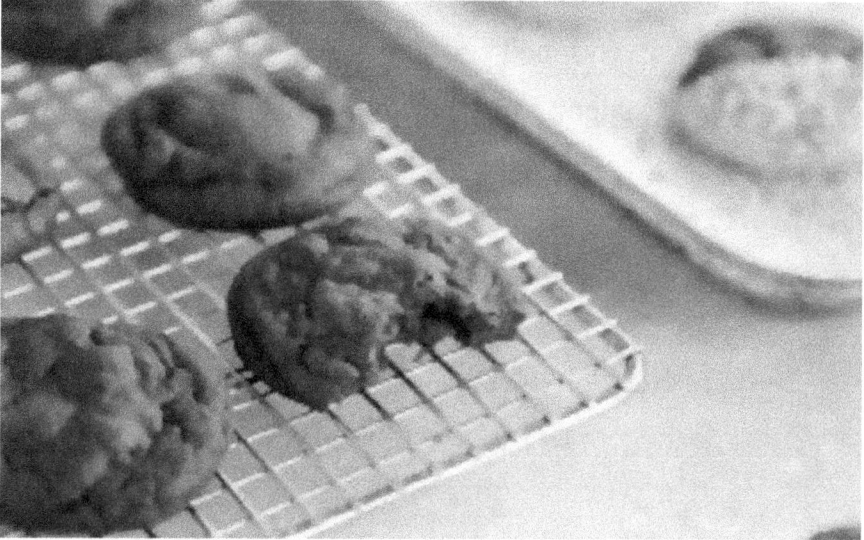

Ingredients:

- 2 tbsp butter, softened
- 1 egg, room temperature
- 1 tbsp Truvia
- ¼ cup Swerve
- 1/8 tsp blackstrap molasses
- 1 tbsp VitaFiber syrup
- 1 tsp vanilla extract
- 6 tbsp sugar-free chocolate chips
- 1 tsp butter
- 6 tbsp almond flour
- 1 tbsp cocoa powder
- 1/8 tsp baking powder

- 1/8 tsp salt
- ¼ tsp xanthan gum
- ¼ cup chopped pecans
- 1 tbsp sugar-free chocolate chips

How to Prepare:

1. Beat egg with 2 tablespoons butter, VitaFiber, sweeteners, and vanilla in a bowl with a hand mixer.
2. Melt ½ of a tablespoon of the chocolate chips with 1 teaspoon of butter in a bowl by heating them in the microwave for 30 seconds then stir well.
3. Add this mixture to the first butter mixture and mix well until smooth.
4. Stir in all the dry ingredients and mix until smooth.
5. Fold in remaining chocolate chips and pecans.
6. Place this batter in the freezer for 8 minutes.
7. Let your oven preheat at 350 degrees F.
8. Grease a baking sheet and drop batter scoop by scoop onto it to form small cookies.
9. Flatten the cookies lightly then bake for 10 minutes.
10. Allow the cookies to cool for about 15 minutes then serve.

Prep Time: 10 minutes

Cooking Time: 12 minutes

Total Time: 22 minutes

Servings: 12

Nutritional Values:

- *Calories 288*
- *Total Fat 25.3 g*
- *Saturated Fat 6.7 g*
- *Cholesterol 23 mg*
- *Sodium 74 mg*
- *Total Carbs 9.6 g*
- *Sugar 0.1 g*
- *Fiber 3.8 g*
- *Protein 7.6 g*

Almond Butter Cookies

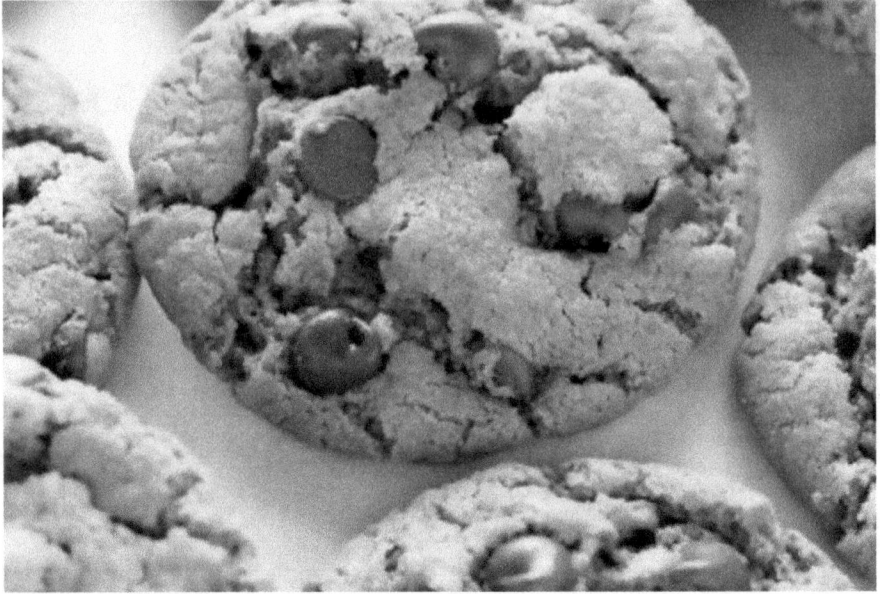

Ingredients:

- 1 cup smooth almond butter
- 4 tbsp unsweetened cocoa powder
- ½ cup granulated erythritol sweetener
- ¼ cup sugar-free chocolate chips
- 1 large egg
- 3 tbsp almond milk unsweetened, if needed

How to Prepare:

1. Preheat your oven at 350 degrees F.
2. Whisk almond butter together with granulated sweetener, egg, and cocoa powder in a bowl with a

fork. Add 3 tbsp almond milk if the mixture is too crumbly.

3. Fold in chocolate chips then make 6-centimeterround cookie balls out of it.

4. Place the balls on a baking sheet lined with parchment paper.

5. Bake them for 12 minutes then allow them to cool.

6. Enjoy.

Prep Time: 5 minutes
Cooking Time: 12 minutes
Total Time: 17 minutes
Servings: 14

Nutritional Values:

- *Calories 77.8*
- *Total Fat 7.13 g*
- *Saturated Fat 4.5 g*
- *Cholesterol 15 mg*
- *Sodium 15 mg*
- *Total Carbs 0.8 g*
- *Sugar 0.2 g*
- *Fiber 0.3 g*
- *Protein 2.3 g*

Macadamia Nut Cookies

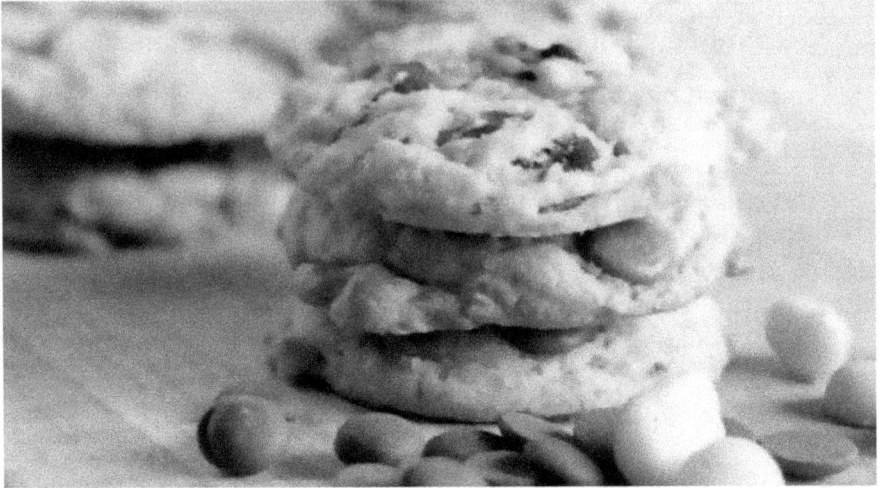

Ingredients:

- ½ cup butter, melted
- 2 tbsp almond butter
- 1 egg
- 1 ½ cup almond flour
- 2 tbsp unsweetened cocoa powder
- ½ cup granulated erythritol sweetener
- 1 tsp vanilla extract
- ½ tsp baking soda
- ¼ cup chopped macadamia nuts
- Pinch of salt

How to Prepare:

1. Preheat your oven to 350 degrees F.

2. Whisk all the ingredients well in a bowl with a fork until smooth.

3. Layer a cookie sheet with wax paper and drop the dough onto it scoop by scoop.

4. Flatten each scoop into 1.5-inch wide round.

5. Bake them for 15 minutes then allow them to cool.

6. Enjoy.

Prep Time: 10 minutes
Cooking Time: 15 minutes
Total Time: 25 minutes
Servings: 12

Nutritional Values:

- *Calories 114*
- *Total Fat 9.6 g*
- *Saturated Fat 4.5 g*
- *Cholesterol 10 mg*
- *Sodium 155 mg*
- *Total Carbs 3.1 g*
- *Sugar 1.4 g*
- *Fiber 1.5 g*
- *Protein 3.5 g*

Chapter 5 Keto Buns and Muffins

Cinnamon Roll Muffins

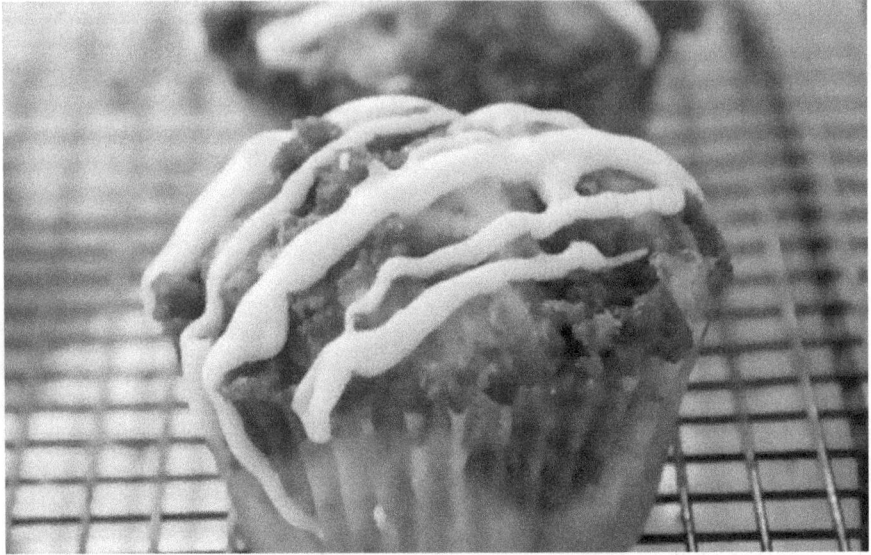

Ingredients:

- ½ cup almond flour
- 2 scoops vanilla protein powder
- 1 tsp baking powder
- 1 tbsp cinnamon
- ½ cup almond butter
- ½ cup pumpkin puree
- ½ cup coconut oil

For the Glaze

- ¼ cup coconut butter
- ¼ cup milk of choice
- 1 tbsp granulated sweetener
- 2 tsp lemon juice

How to Prepare:

1. Let your oven preheat at 350 degrees F. Layer a 12-cup muffin tray with muffin liners.
2. Add all the dry ingredients to a suitable mixing bowl then whisk in all the wet ingredients.
3. Mix until well combined then divide the batter into the muffin cups.
4. Bake them for 15 minutes then allow the muffins to cool on a wire rack.
5. Prepare the cinnamon glaze in a small bowl then drizzle this glaze over the muffins.
6. Enjoy.

Prep Time: 5 minutes
Cooking Time: 15 minutes
Total Time: 20 minutes
Servings: 6

Nutritional Values:

- *Calories 252*
- *Total Fat 17.3 g*
- *Saturated Fat 11.5 g*
- *Cholesterol 141 mg*
- *Sodium 153 mg*
- *Total Carbs 7.2 g*
- *Sugar 0.3 g*
- *Fiber 1.4 g*
- *Protein 5.2 g*

Muffins with Blueberries

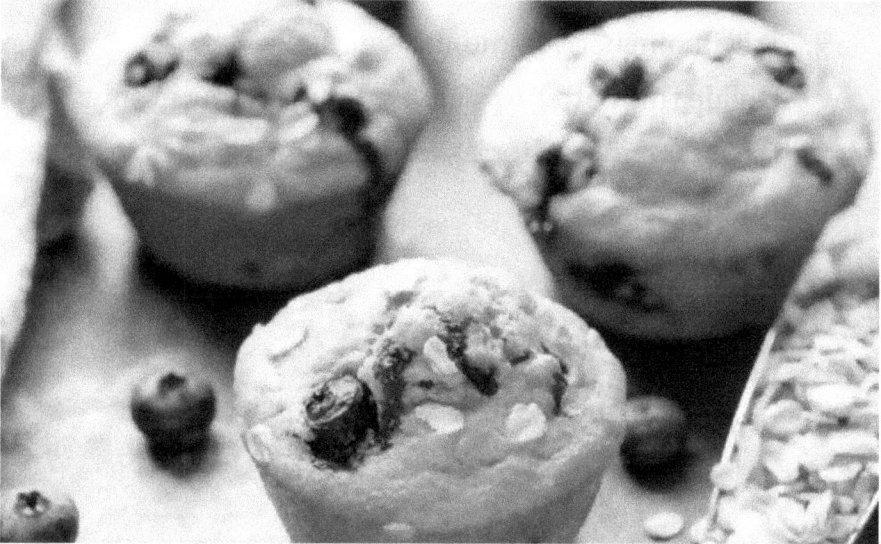

Ingredients:

- ¾ cup coconut flour
- 6 eggs
- ½ cup coconut oil, melted
- 1/3 cup unsweetened coconut milk
- ½ cup fresh blueberries
- 1/3 cup granulated sweetener
- 1 tsp vanilla extract
- 1 tsp baking powder

How to Prepare:

1. Preheat your oven at 356 degrees F.

2. Mix coconut flour with all the other ingredients except blueberries in a mixing bowl until smooth.
3. Stir in blueberries and mix gently.
4. Divide this batter in a greased muffin tray evenly.
5. Bake the muffins for 25 minutes until golden brown.
6. Enjoy.

Prep Time: 10 minutes
Cooking Time: 25 minutes
Total Time: 35 minutes
Servings: 8

Nutritional Values:

- *Calories 195*
- *Total Fat 14.3 g*
- *Saturated Fat 10.5 g*
- *Cholesterol 175 mg*
- *Sodium 125 mg*
- *Total Carbs 4.5 g*
- *Sugar 0.5 g*
- *Fiber 0.3 g*
- *Protein 3.2 g*

Chocolate Zucchini Muffins

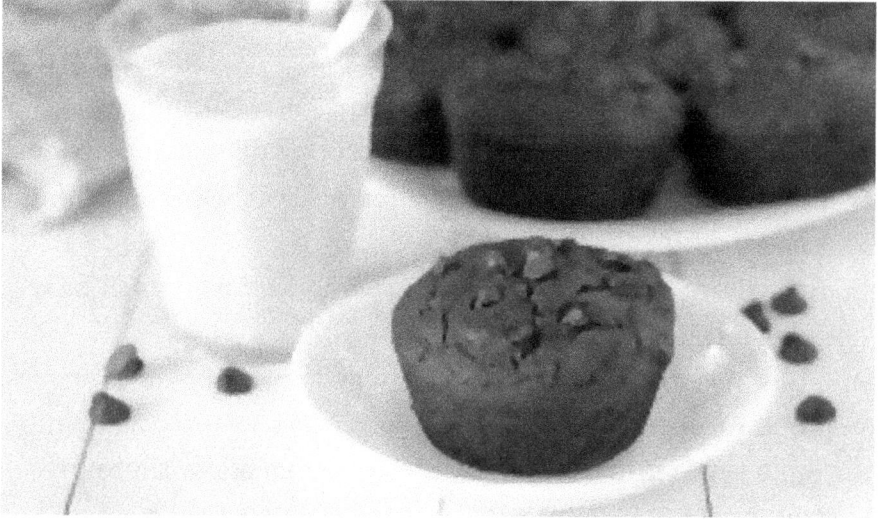

Ingredients:

- ½ cup coconut flour
- ¾ tsp baking soda
- 2 tbsp cocoa powder
- ½ tsp salt
- 1 tsp cinnamon
- ½ tsp nutmeg
- 3 large eggs
- 2/3 cup Swerve sweetener
- 2 tsp vanilla extract
- 1 tbsp oil
- 1 medium zucchini, grated
- ¼ cup heavy cream
- 1/3 cup Lily's chocolate baking chips

How to Prepare:

1. Preheat your oven at 356 degrees F.
2. Layer a 9-cup o muffin tray with muffin liners then spray them with cooking oil.
3. Whisk coconut flour with salt, cinnamon, nutmeg, sweetener, baking soda, and cocoa powder in a bowl.
4. Beat eggs in a separate bowl then add oil, cream, vanilla, and zucchini.
5. Stir in the coconut flour mixture and mix well until fully incorporated.
6. Fold in chocolate chips then divide the batter into the lined muffin cups.
7. Bake these muffins for 30 minutes then allow them to cool on a wire rack.
8. Enjoy.

Prep Time: 10 minutes
Cooking Time: 30 minutes
Total Time: 40 minutes
Servings: 9

Nutritional Values:

- *Calories 151*
- *Total Fat 14.7 g*
- *Saturated Fat 1.5 g*
- *Cholesterol 13 mg*
- *Sodium 53 mg*
- *Total Carbs 1.5 g*
- *Sugar 0.3 g*
- *Fiber 0.1 g*
- *Protein 0.8 g*

Blackberry-Filled Lemon Muffins

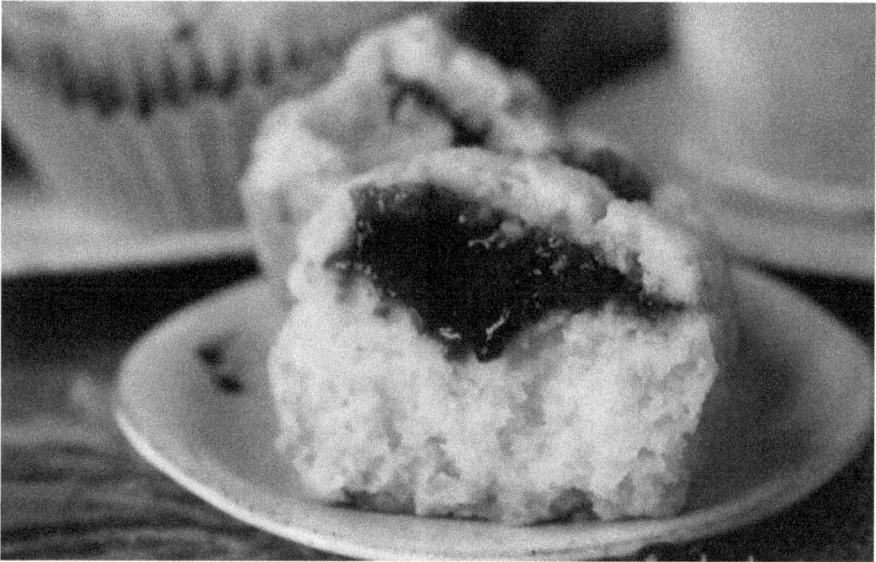

Ingredients:

For the Blackberry Filling:
- 3 tbsp granulated stevia
- 1 tsp lemon juice
- ¼ tsp xanthan gum
- 2 tbsp water
- 1 cup fresh blackberries

For the Muffin Batter:
- 2 ½ cups super fine almond flour
- ¾ cup granulasted stevia
- 1 tsp fresh lemon zest

- ½ tsp sea salt
- 1 tsp grain-free baking powder
- 4 large eggs
- ¼ cup unsweetened almond milk
- ¼ cup butter
- 1 tsp vanilla extract
- ½ tsp lemon extract

How to Prepare:

For the Blackberry Filling:
1. Add granulated sweetener and xanthan gum in a saucepan.
2. Stir in lemon juice and water then place it over the medium heat.
3. Add blackberries and stir cook on low heat for 10 minutes.
4. Remove the saucepan from the heat and allow the mixture to cool.

For the Muffin Batter:
5. Preheat your oven at 356 degrees F and layer a muffin tray with paper cups.
6. Mix almond flour with salt, baking powder, lemon zest, baking powder, and sweetener in a mixing bowl.
7. Whisk in eggs, vanilla extract, lemon extract, butter, and almond milk.

8. Beat well until smooth. Divide half of this batter into the muffin tray.
9. Make a depression at the center of each muffin.
10. Add a spoonful of blackberry jam mixture to each depression.
11. Cover the filling with remaining batter on top.
12. Bake the muffins for 30 minutes then allow them to cool.
13. Refrigerate for a few hours before serving.
14. Enjoy.

Prep Time: 5 minutes
Cooking Time: 30 minutes
Total Time: 35 minutes
Servings: 12

Nutritional Values:
- *Calories 261*
- *Total Fat 7.1 g*
- *Saturated Fat 13.4 g*
- *Cholesterol 0.3 mg*
- *Sodium 10 mg*
- *Total Carbs 6.1 g*
- *Sugar 2.1 g*
- *Fiber 3.9 g*
- *Protein 1.8 g*

Banana Muffins

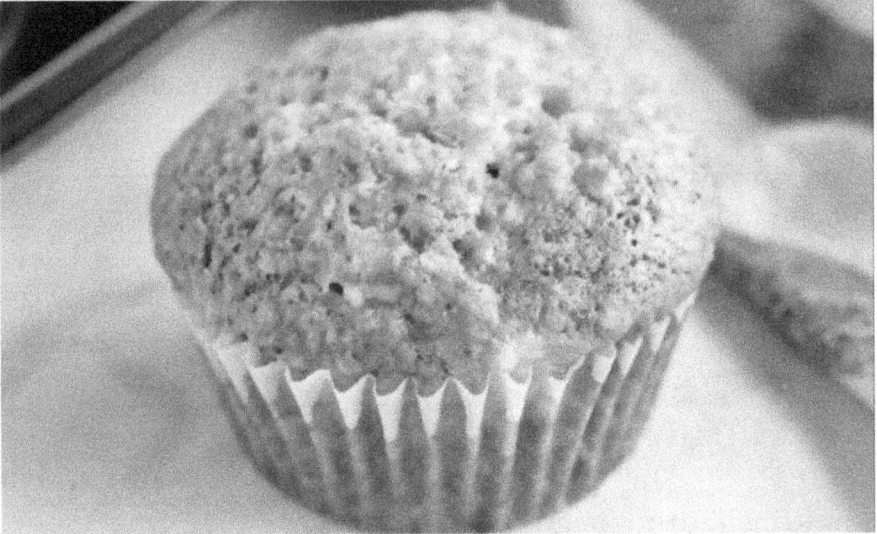

Ingredients:

- 3 large eggs
- 2 cups bananas, mashed (3-4 medium bananas)
- ½ cup almond butter (peanut butter can also be used)
- ¼ cup butter (olive oil can also be used)
- 1 tsp vanilla
- ½ cup coconut flour (almond flour can also be used)
- 1 tbsp cinnamon
- 1 tsp baking powder
- 1 tsp baking soda
- Pinch sea salt
- ½ cup chocolate chips

How to Prepare:

1. Preheat your oven at 356 degrees F.
2. Line a 12-cup muffin tray with paper liners.
3. Whisk eggs with almond butter, vanilla, butter, and mashed bananas in a large bowl.
4. Stir in coconut flour, baking soda, cinnamon, baking powder, and salt. Mix well with a wooden spoon.
5. Divide this batter into the muffin cups then bake them for 18 minutes.
6. Allow them to cool then refrigerate for 30 minutes.
7. Enjoy.

Prep Time: 10 minutes
Cooking Time: 18 minutes
Total Time: 28 minutes
Servings: 12

Nutritional Values:

- *Calories 139*
- *Total Fat 4.6 g*
- *Saturated Fat 0.5 g*
- *Cholesterol 1.2 mg*
- *Sodium 83 mg*
- *Total Carbs 7.5 g*
- *Sugar 6.3 g*
- *Fiber 0.6 g*
- *Protein 3.8 g*

Breakfast Buns

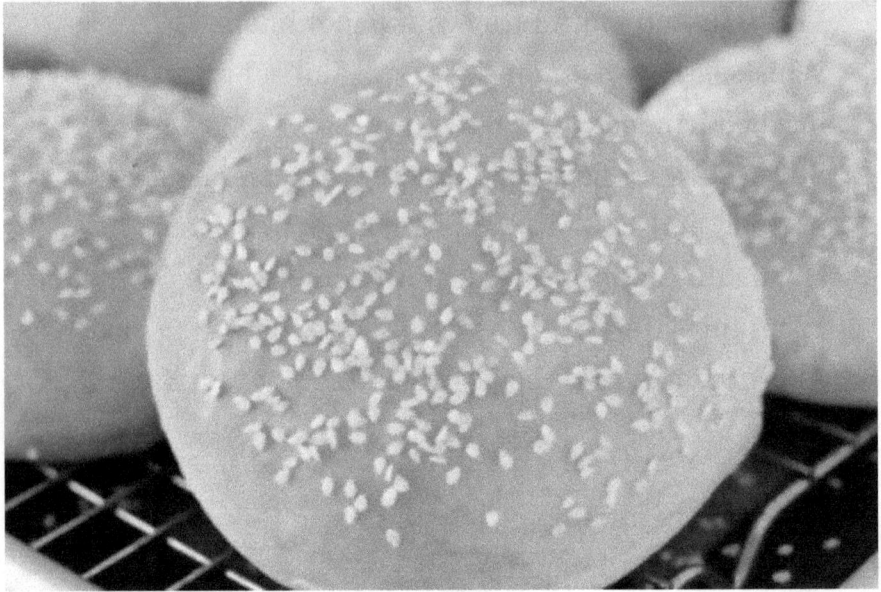

Ingredients:

- 3 egg whites, room temperature
- 1 egg, room temperature
- ¼ cup boiling hot water
- ¼ cup almond flour
- ¼ cup coconut flour
- 1 tbsp psyllium husk powder
- 1 tsp baking powder
- Sesame seeds, for sprinkling

How to Prepare:

1. Preheat your oven at 356 degrees F.

2. Add everything to a food processor and blend for 20 seconds until smooth.
3. Let it sit for 20 minutes then divide the dough into 4 equal parts.
4. Shape the dough into buns then place them on a baking sheet lined with wax paper.
5. Score the top of each bun with a fork and sprinkle sesame seeds on top.
6. Bake the buns for 25 minutes until golden brown.
7. Enjoy.

Prep Time: 10 minutes
Cooking Time: 25 minutes
Total Time: 35 minutes
Servings: 4

Nutritional Values:
- *Calories 200*
- *Total Fat 11.1 g*
- *Saturated Fat 9.5 g*
- *Cholesterol 124.2 mg*
- *Sodium 46 mg*
- *Total Carbs 1.1 g*
- *Sugar 1.3 g*
- *Fiber 0.4 g*
- *Protein 0.4 g*

Dinner Rolls

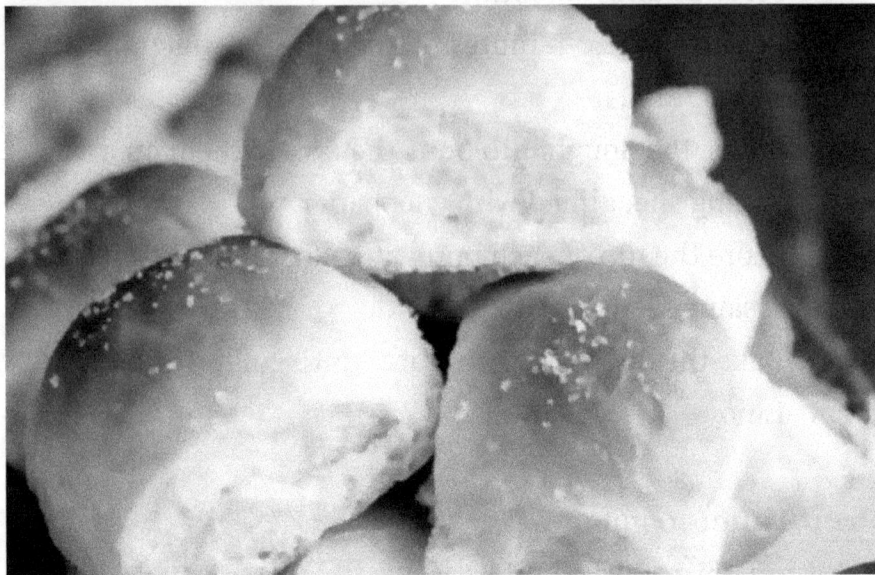

Ingredients:
- 1 cup mozzarella, shredded
- 1 oz cream cheese
- 1 cup almond flour
- ¼ cup ground flaxseed
- 1 egg
- ½ tsp baking soda

How to Prepare:
1. Preheat your oven at 400 degrees F.
2. Layer a baking sheet with wax paper and set it aside.
3. Melt mozzarella and cream cheese in a medium bowl by heating the mixture for 1 minute in the microwave.
4. Mix well then add the egg. Whisk well until combined.

5. Add baking soda, flaxseed, and almond flour.
6. Mix well to form a smooth dough then make 6 balls out of this dough.
7. Place the balls on the baking sheet lined with wax paper.
8. Sprinkle sesame seeds over the balls.
9. Bake them for 12 minutes until golden brown.
10. Enjoy.

Prep Time: 5 minutes
Cooking Time: 12 minutes
Total Time: 17 minutes
Servings: 8

Nutritional Values:
- *Calories 136*
- *Total Fat 10.7 g*
- *Saturated Fat 0.5 g*
- *Cholesterol 4 mg*
- *Sodium 45 mg*
- *Total Carbs 1.2 g*
- *Sugar 1.4 g*
- *Fiber 0.2 g*
- *Protein 0.9*

Buns with Psyllium Husk

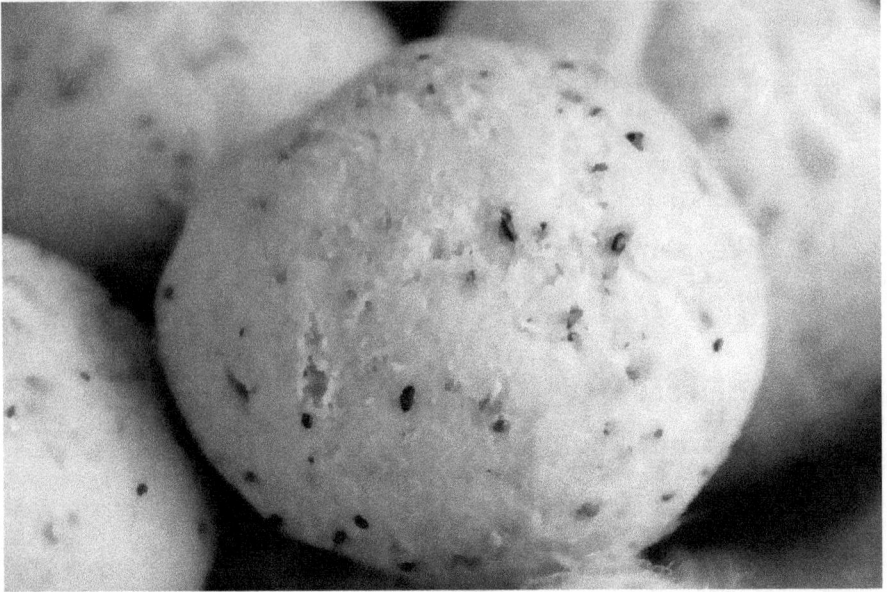

Ingredients:

- 4 tbsp boiling water

Dry Ingredients

- 3.53 oz blanched almond flour
- 2 tbsp psyllium husk powder
- 1 tsp baking powder
- 1 tsp black sesame seeds
- 1 tsp white sesame seeds
- 2 tsp sunflower seeds
- 1 tsp black chia seeds

- ½ tsp Himalayan salt
- ½ tsp garlic powder

Wet Ingredients

- 1 egg
- 2 egg whites
- 1 tbsp apple cider vinegar
- 3 tbsp melted refined coconut oil

How to Prepare:

1. Preheat your oven at 356 degrees F.
2. Add dry ingredients to a bowl along with wet ingredients. Mix well until smooth.
3. Slowly add boiled water into the dough and mix well to absorb the water.
4. Divide the dough into 5 balls, grease them with cooking oil.and roll them in your hands.
5. Place the balls on a baking sheet lined with parchment paper.
6. Bake them for 30 minutes until golden.
7. Enjoy.

Prep Time: 15 minutes

Cooking Time: 30 minutes

Total Time: 45 minutes

Servings: 5

Nutritional Values:

- *Calories 76*
- *Total Fat 7.2 g*
- *Saturated Fat 6.4 g*
- *Cholesterol 134 mg*
- *Sodium 8 mg*
- *Total Carbs 2g*
- *Sugar 1 g*
- *Fiber 0.7 g*
- *Protein 2.2 g*

Fathead Rolls

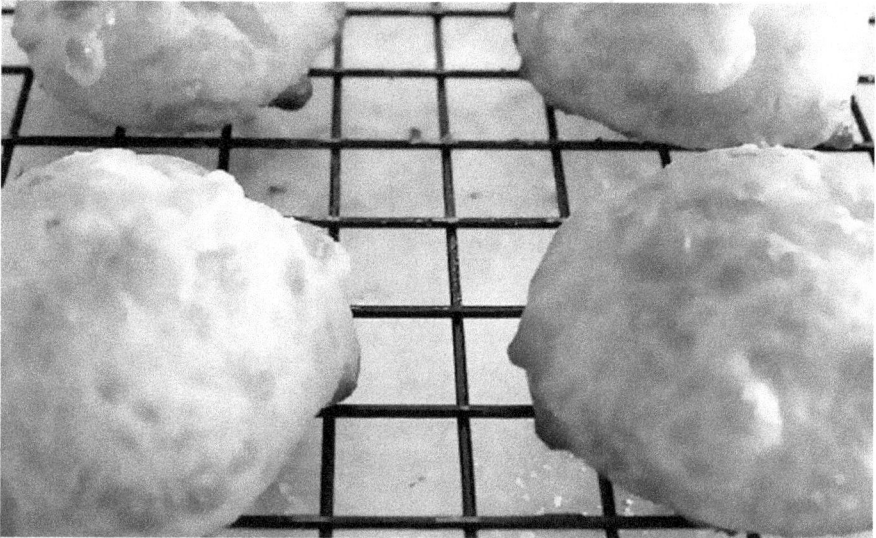

Ingredients:
- 2 oz cream cheese
- ¾ cup shredded mozzarella
- 1 egg beaten
- ¼ tsp garlic powder
- 1/3 cup almond flour
- 2 tsp baking powder
- ½ cup shredded cheddar cheese

How to Prepare:
1. Preheat your oven at 425 degrees F.
2. Heat mozzarella and cream cheese in a small bowl for 20 seconds in the microwave.
3. Beat egg with all the dry ingredients in a separate bowl.

4. Stir in cheese mixture to make a sticky dough adding the cheddar cheese at the end.
5. Mix well then wrap the dough in plastic wrap.
6. Refrigerate this dough for 30 minutes then divide it into 4 equal parts.
7. Cut each ball in half and place them flat side down on a baking sheet lined with wax paper.
8. Bake them for 12 minutes until golden.
9. Enjoy.

Prep Time: 5 minutes
Cooking Time: 12 minutes
Total Time: 17 minutes
Servings: 6

Nutritional Values:
- *Calories 193*
- *Total Fat 10 g*
- *Saturated Fat 13.2 g*
- *Cholesterol 120 mg*
- *Sodium 8 mg*
- *Total Carbs 2.5 g*
- *Sugar 1 g*
- *Fiber 0.7 g*
- *Protein 2.2 g*

Chapter 6 Keto Fat Bombs

Vanilla Cheesecake Fat Bombs

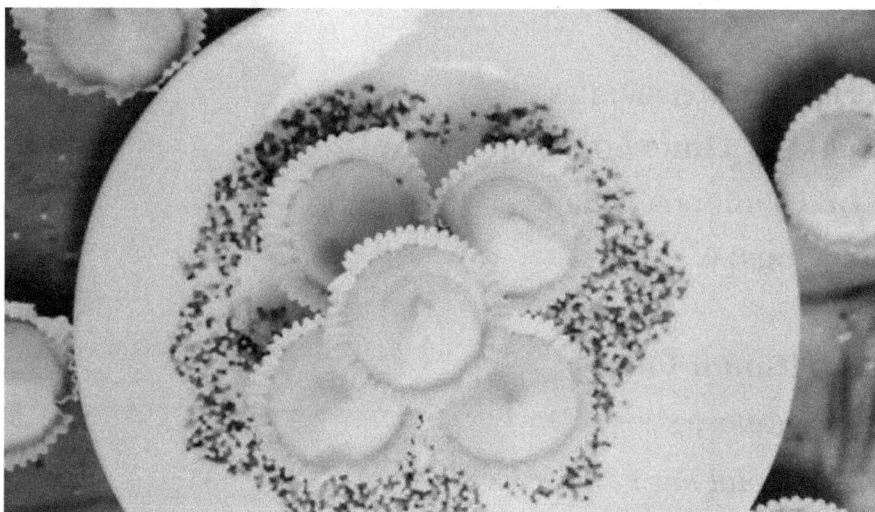

Ingredients:

- 9 oz cream cheese, softened
- 2 tsp vanilla extract
- 2 oz erythritol
- 1 cup heavy cream

How to Prepare:

1. In a bowl, mix erythritol, vanilla, and cream cheese with a hand mixer on low speed for two minutes.
2. Slowly add heavy cream to the mixture while beating it continuously until it forms peaks.

3. Divide the mixture into a muffin tray layered with cupcake liners.
4. Place this tray in the refrigerator for 1 hour to set.
5. Enjoy.

Prep Time: 5 minutes
Cooking Time: 60 minutes
Total Time: 65 minutes
Servings: 6

Nutritional Values:
- *Calories 173*
- *Total Fat 13 g*
- *Saturated Fat 10.1 g*
- *Cholesterol 12 mg*
- *Sodium 67 mg*
- *Total Carbs 7.5 g*
- *Sugar 1.2 g*
- *Fiber 0.6 g*
- *Protein 3.2 g*

Raspberry Cream Fat Bombs

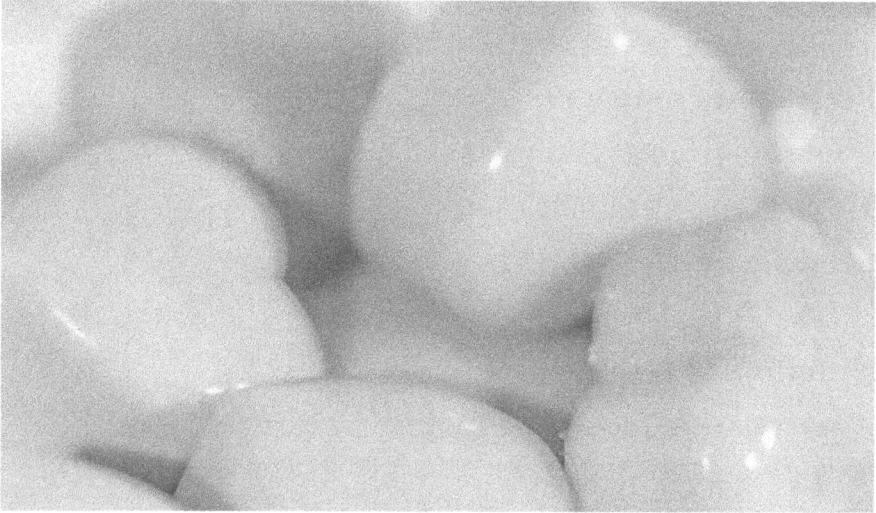

Ingredients:

- 1 packet raspberry Jello (sugar-free)
- 1 tsp gelatin powder
- ½ cup of boiling water
- ½ cup heavy cream

How to Prepare:

1. Mix Jello and gelatin in boiling water in a medium bowl.
2. Stir in cream slowly and mix it for 1 minute.
3. Divide this mixture into candy molds.

4. Refrigerate them for 30 minutes.
5. Enjoy.

Prep Time: 5 minutes
Cooking Time: 30 minutes
Total Time: 35 minutes
Servings: 13

Nutritional Values:

- *Calories 197*
- *Total Fat 19.2 g*
- *Saturated Fat 10.1 g*
- *Cholesterol 11 mg*
- *Sodium 78 mg*
- *Total Carbs 7.3 g*
- *Sugar 1.2 g*
- *Fiber 0.8 g*
- *Protein 4.2 g*

Red Velvet Fat Bombs

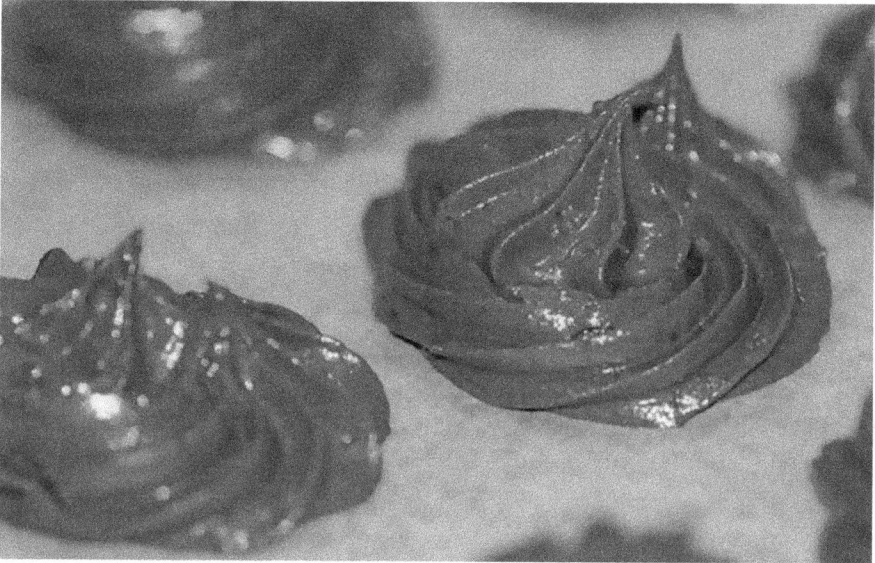

Ingredients:

- ¼ cup 90% dark chocolate
- 1/3 cup cream cheese, softened
- ¼ cup butter, softened
- 3 tbsp natvia sweetener
- 1 tsp vanilla extract
- 4 drops red food coloring
- 1/3 cup heavy cream, whipped

How to Prepare:

1. Add chocolate to a heatproof bowl and melt it in a microwave for 1 minute.

2. Whisk cream cheese with butter, natvia, vanilla extract, and food coloring in a bowl using a hand mixer until fluffy.
3. Slowly stir in the melted chocolate while beating the mixture with the hand mixer on medium speed.
4. After 2 minutes of beating, transfer the mixture to a piping bag.
5. Pipe the mixture onto a baking sheet lined with baking paper to make small fat bombs.
6. Place them in the refrigerator for 40 minutes.
7. Garnish the fat bombs with heavy cream.
8. Serve.

Prep Time: 5 minutes
Cooking Time: 40 minutes
Total Time: 45 minutes
Servings: 12

Nutritional Values:
- *Calories 213*
- *Total Fat 19 g*
- *Saturated Fat 15.2 g*
- *Cholesterol 13 mg*
- *Sodium 52 mg*
- *Total Carbs 5.5 g*
- *Sugar 1.3 g*
- *Fiber 0.5 g*
- *Protein 6.1 g*

Pina Colada Fat Bombs

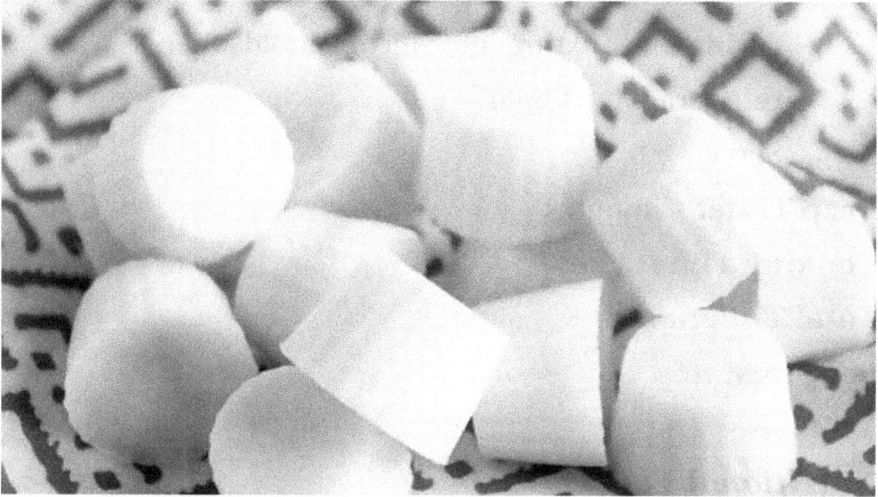

Ingredients:

- 2 tsp pineapple essence
- 3 tsp erythritol
- 2 tbsp gelatin
- ½ cup boiling water
- ½ cup coconut cream
- 1 tsp rum extract
- 2 scoops MCT powder

How to Prepare:

1. Mix gelatin with boiling water and erythritol in a bowl.
2. Add pineapple essence and mix well then let it sit for 5 minutes.

3. Stir in coconut cream and rum extract then stir this mixture for 2 minutes.

4. Divide this mixture into silicone molds then refrigerate for 1 hour.

5. Serve.

Prep Time: 5 minutes

Cooking Time: 1 hour

Total Time: 1 hour & 5 minutes

Servings: 16

Nutritional Values:

- *Calories 117*
- *Total Fat 21.2 g*
- *Saturated Fat 10.4 g*
- *Cholesterol 19.7 mg*
- *Sodium 104 mg*
- *Total Carbs 7.3 g*
- *Sugar 3.4 g*
- *Fiber 2 g*
- *Protein 8.1 g*

Lemon and Poppy Seed Fat Bombs

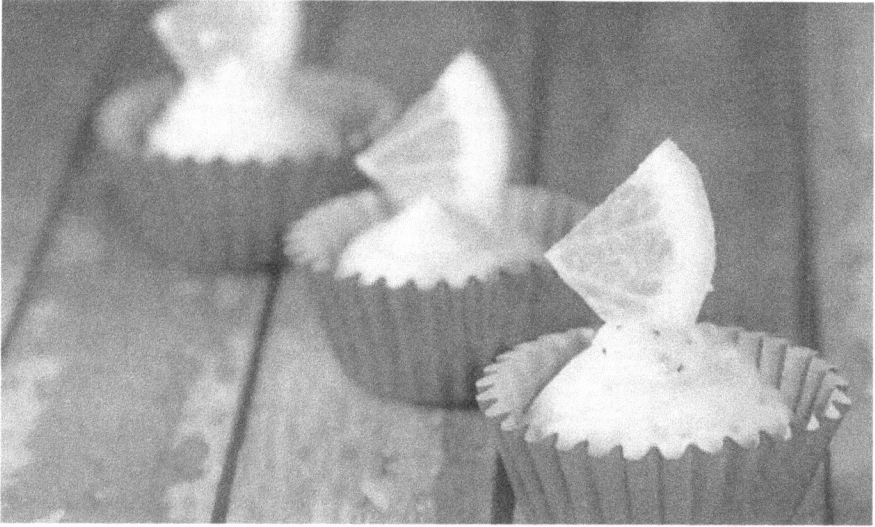

Ingredients:

- 8 oz cream cheese, softened
- 3 tbsp erythritol
- 1 tbsp poppy seeds
- 1 lemon, zested
- 4 tbsp sour cream
- 2 tbsp lemon juice

How to Prepare:

1. Add everything to a bowl and beat them together using a hand mixer on low speed for 3 minutes.

2. Divide this mixture into a mini cupcake tray layered with cupcake liners and place it in the refrigerator for 1 hour.
3. Serve.

Prep Time: 5 minutes
Cooking Time: 1 hour
Total Time: 1 hour & 5 minutes
Servings: 18

Nutritional Values:

- Calories 113
- Total Fat 9 g
- Saturated Fat 0.2 g
- Cholesterol 1.7 mg
- Sodium 134 mg
- Total Carbs 6.5 g
- Sugar 1.8 g
- Fiber 0.7 g
- Protein 7.5 g

Chapter 7 Keto Snacks and Treats

Peanut Butter Granola

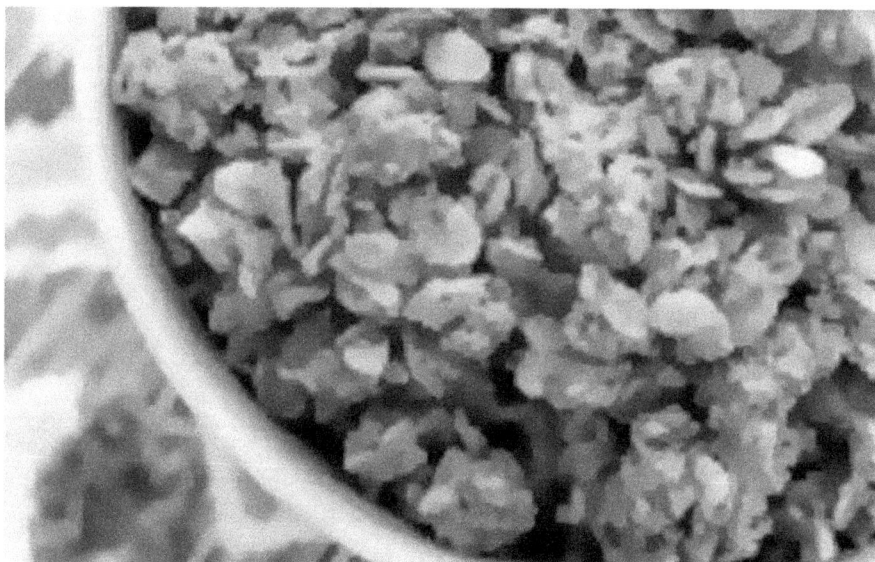

Ingredients:

- 1 ½ cups almonds

- 1 ½ cups pecans

- 1 cup shredded coconut

- ¼ cup sunflower seeds

- 1/3 cup Swerve sweetener

- 1/3 cup vanilla whey protein powder

- 1/3 cup peanut butter

- ¼ cup butter
- ¼ cup water

How to Prepare:

1. Preheat your oven at 300 degrees F.
2. Layer a baking sheet with wax paper and set it aside.
3. Add almonds and pecans to a food processor and finely grind them.
4. Add coconut, protein powder, sweetener, and sunflower seeds to the nut mixture in a bowl.
5. Add butter and peanut butter to another bowl and melt it in the microwave by heating for 30 sec or 1 minute.
6. Mix well then pour it into the nut mixture.
7. After mixing it up, spread this mixture on a baking sheet in an even layer.
8. Bake for 30 minutes then allow it to cool.
9. Serve.

Prep Time: 5 minutes

Cooking Time: 30 minutes

Total Time: 35 minutes

Servings: 12

Nutritional Values:

- *Calories 101*
- *Total Fat 15.5 g*
- *Saturated Fat 4.5 g*
- *Cholesterol 12 mg*
- *Sodium 18 mg*
- *Total Carbs 4.4 g*
- *Sugar 1.2 g*
- *Fiber 0.3 g*
- *Protein 4.8 g*

Blueberry Scones

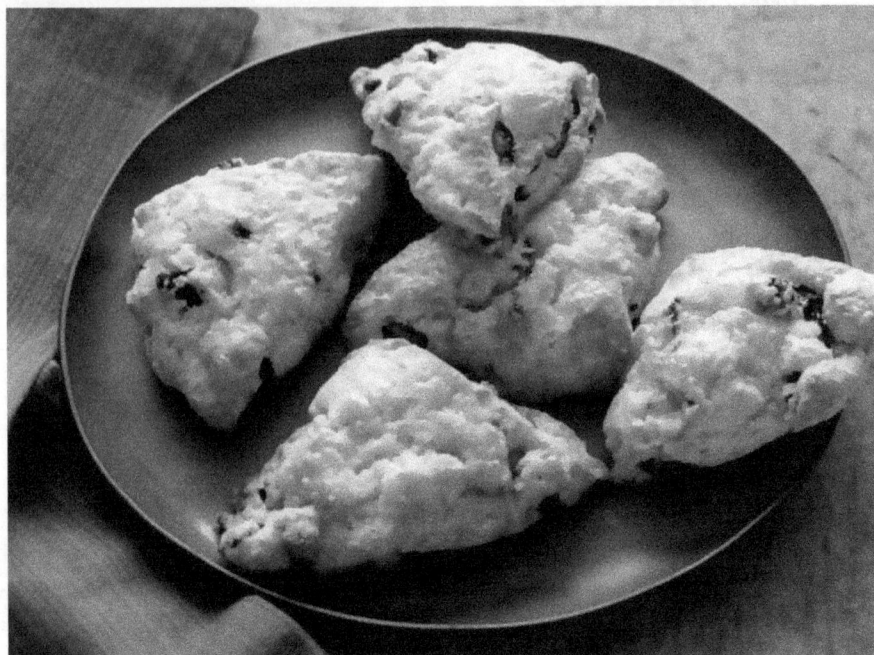

Ingredients:

- 2 cups almond flour
- 1/3 cup Swerve sweetener
- ¼ cup coconut flour
- 1 tbsp baking powder
- ¼ tsp salt
- 2 large eggs
- ¼ cup heavy whipping cream
- ½ tsp vanilla extract
- ¾ cup fresh blueberries

How to Prepare:

1. Preheat your oven at 325 degrees F. Layer a baking sheet with wax paper.

2. Whisk almond flour with baking powder, salt, coconut flour, and sweetener in a large bowl.

3. Stir in eggs, vanilla, and cream then mix well until fully incorporated.

4. Add blueberries and mix gently.

5. Spread this dough on a baking sheet and form it into a 10x8-inch rectangle.

6. Slice the dough into 6 equal-sized squares then cut each diagonally to make triangles.

7. Arrange these triangles on the baking sheet 1 inch apart from each other.

8. Bake these scones for 25 minutes until golden.

9. Allow them to cool then serve.

Prep Time: 5 minutes

Cooking Time: 25 minutes

Total Time: 30 minutes

Servings: 12

Nutritional Values:

- *Calories 266*
- *Total Fat 25.7 g*
- *Saturated Fat 1.2 g*
- *Cholesterol 41 mg*
- *Sodium 18 mg*
- *Total Carbs 9.7 g*
- *Sugar 1.2 g*
- *Fiber 0.5 g*
- *Protein 2.6 g*

Homemade Graham Crackers

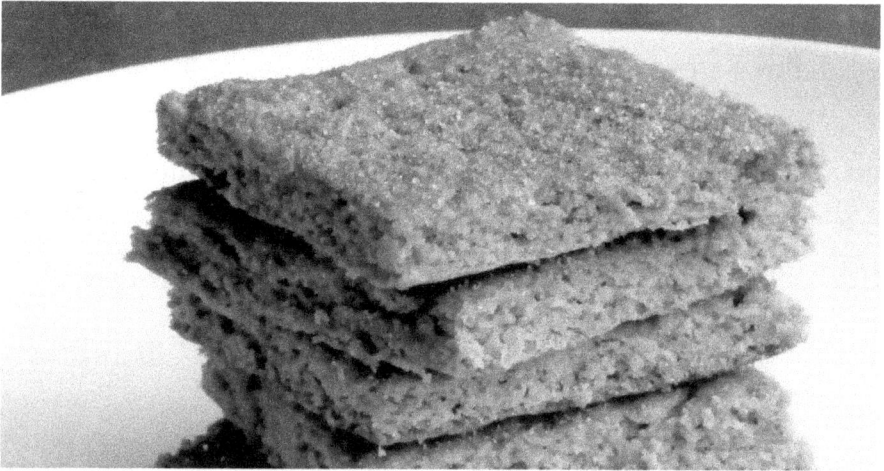

Ingredients:
- 2 cups almond flour
- 1/3 cup Swerve Brown
- 2 tsp cinnamon
- 1 tsp baking powder
- Pinch salt
- 1 large egg
- 2 tbsp butter, melted
- 1 tsp vanilla extract

How to Prepare:
1. Preheat your oven at 300 degrees F.
2. Whisk almond flour, baking powder, salt, cinnamon, and sweetener in a large bowl.
3. Stir in melted butter, egg, and vanilla extract.

4. Mix well to form the dough then spread it out into a ¼-inch thick sheet.
5. Slice the sheet into 2x2-inch squares and place them on a baking sheet with wax paper.
6. Bake them for 30 minutes until golden then let them sit for 30 minutes at room temperature until cooled.
7. Break the crackers into smaller squares and put them back in the hot oven for 30 minutes. Keep the oven off during this time.
8. Enjoy.

Prep Time: 5 minutes
Cooking Time: 30 minutes
Total Time: 35 minutes
Servings: 12

Nutritional Values:
- *Calories 243*
- *Total Fat 21 g*
- *Saturated Fat 18.2 g*
- *Cholesterol 121 mg*
- *Sodium 34 mg*
- *Total Carbs 7.3 g*
- *Sugar 0.9 g*
- *Fiber 0.1 g*
- *Protein 4.3 g*

Buffalo Chicken Sausage Balls

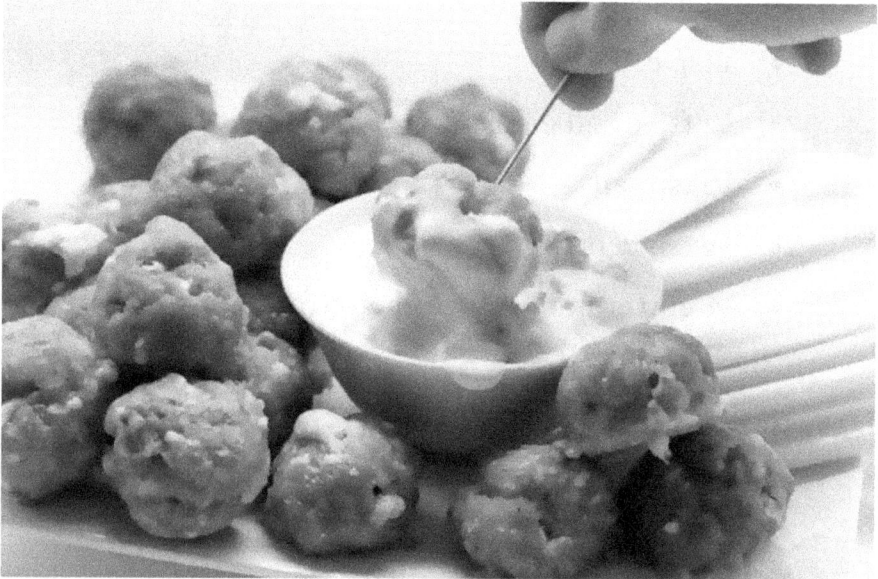

Ingredients:

Sausage Balls:

- 2 14-ox sausages, casings removed
- 2 cups almond flour
- 1 ½ cups shredded cheddar cheese
- ½ cup crumbled bleu cheese
- 1 tsp salt
- ½ tsp pepper

Bleu Cheese Ranch Dipping Sauce:

- 1/3 cup mayonnaise

- 1/3 cup almond milk, unsweetened
- 2 cloves garlic, minced
- 1 tsp dried dill
- ½ tsp dried parsley
- ½ tsp salt
- ½ tsp pepper
- ¼ cup crumbled bleu cheese (or more, if desired)

How to Prepare:

1. Preheat your oven at 350 degrees F.
2. Layer two baking sheets with wax paper and set them aside.
3. Mix sausage with cheddar cheese, almond flour, salt, pepper, and bleu cheese in a large bowl.
4. Make 1-inch balls out of this mixture and place them on the baking sheets.
5. Bake them for 25 minutes until golden brown.
6. Meanwhile, prepare the dipping sauce by whisking all of its ingredients in a bowl.
7. Serve the balls with this dipping sauce.

Prep Time: 5 minutes

Cooking Time: 25 minutes

Total Time: 30 minutes

Servings: 12

Nutritional Values:

- *Calories 183*
- *Total Fat 15 g*
- *Saturated Fat 12.1 g*
- *Cholesterol 11 mg*
- *Sodium 31 mg*
- *Total Carbs 6.2 g*
- *Sugar 1.6 g*
- *Fiber 0.8 g*
- *Protein 4.5 g*

Brussels Sprouts Chips

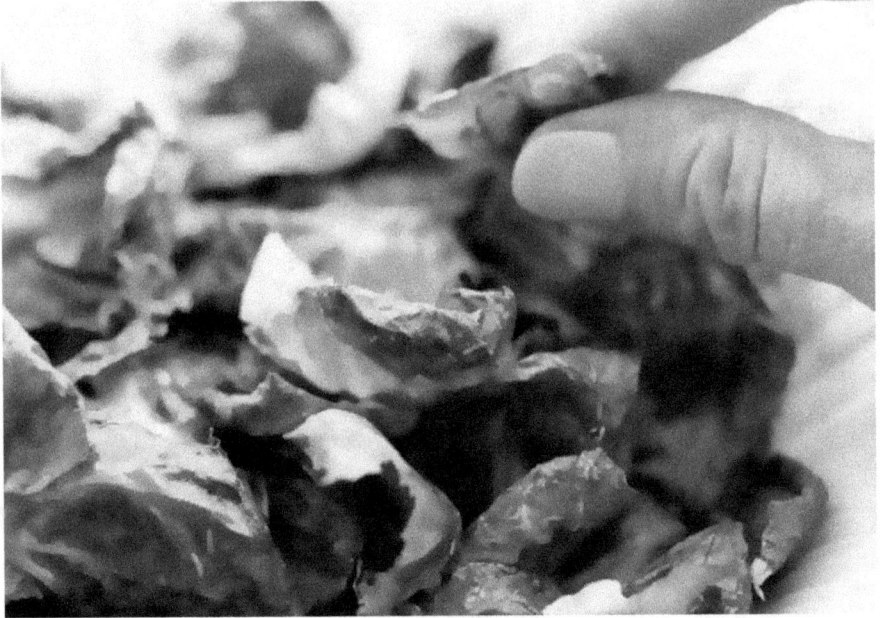

Ingredients:

- 1 pound Brussels sprouts, washed and dried
- 2 tbsp extra virgin olive oil
- 1 tsp kosher salt

How to Prepare:

1. Preheat your oven at 400 degrees F.
2. After peeling the sprouts off the stem, discard the outer leaves of the Brussel sprouts.
3. Separate all the leaves from one another and place them on a baking sheet.

4. Toss them with oil and salt thoroughly to coat them well.
5. Spread the leaves out on two greased baking sheets then bake them for 15 minutes until crispy.
6. Serve.

Prep Time: 5 minutes
Cooking Time: 15 minutes
Total Time: 20 minutes
Servings: 6

Nutritional Values:

- *Calories 188*
- *Total Fat 3 g*
- *Saturated Fat 2.2 g*
- *Cholesterol 101 mg*
- *Sodium 54 mg*
- *Total Carbs 3 g*
- *Sugar 1.3 g*
- *Fiber 0.6 g*
- *Protein 5 g*

Chapter 8 Keto Ice Cream, Pudding, Mousse

Keto Chocolate Mousse

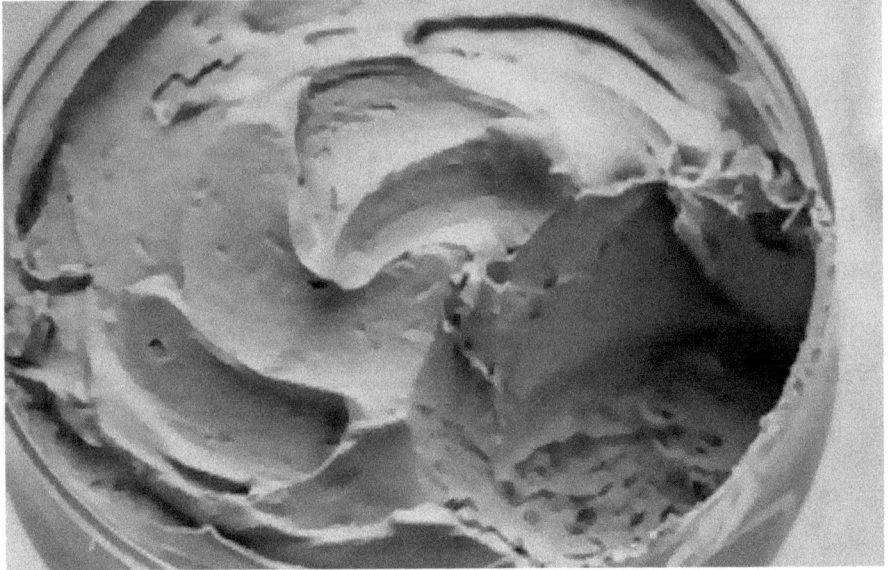

Ingredients:

- 1 cup heavy whipping cream
- ¼ cup unsweetened cocoa powder, sifted
- ¼ cup Swerve powdered sweetener
- 1 tsp vanilla extract
- ¼ tsp kosher salt

How to Prepare:

1. Add cream to the bowl of an electric stand mixture and beat it until it forms peaks.
2. Stir in cocoa powder, vanilla, sweetener, and salt.
3. Mix well until smooth.
4. Refrigerate for 4 hours.
5. Serve.

Prep Time: 5 minutes
Cooking Time: 4 hours
Total Time: 4 hours & 5 minutes
Servings: 2

Nutritional Values:

- *Calories 153*
- *Total Fat 13 g*
- *Saturated Fat 9.2 g*
- *Cholesterol 6.5 mg*
- *Sodium 81 mg*
- *Total Carbs 4.5 g*
- *Sugar 1.4 g*
- *Fiber 0.4 g*
- *Protein 5.8 g*

Keto Berry Mousse

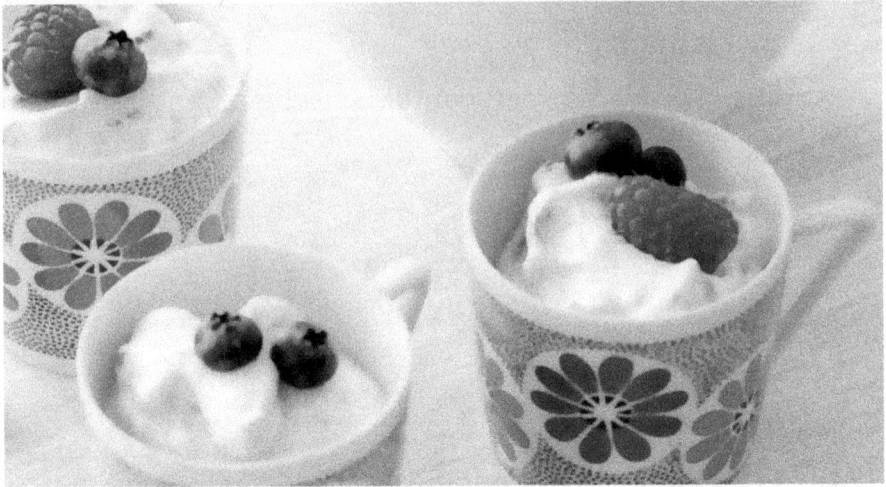

Ingredients:

- 2 cups heavy whipping cream
- 3 oz fresh raspberries
- 2 oz chopped pecans
- ½ lemon, zested
- ¼ tsp vanilla extract

How to Prepare:

1. Beat cream in a bowl using a hand mixer until it forms peaks.
2. Stir in vanilla and lemon zest and mix well until incorporated.
3. Fold in nuts and berries and mix well.

4. Cover the mixture with plastic wrap and refrigerate for 3 hours.
5. Serve fresh.

Prep Time: 5 minutes
Cooking Time: 3 hours
Total Time: 3 hours & 5 minutes
Servings: 2

Nutritional Values:

- *Calories 254*
- *Total Fat 9 g*
- *Saturated Fat 10.1 g*
- *Cholesterol 13 mg*
- *Sodium 179 mg*
- *Total Carbs 7.5 g*
- *Sugar 1.2 g*
- *Fiber 0.8 g*
- *Protein 7.5 g*

Peanut Butter Mousse

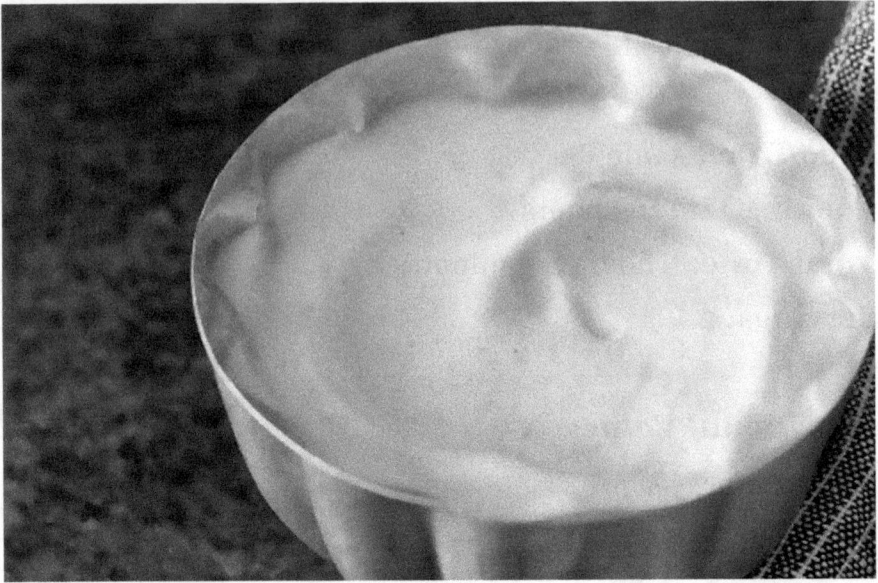

Ingredients:

- ½ cup heavy whipping cream
- 4 oz cream cheese, softened
- ¼ cup natural peanut butter
- ¼ cup powdered Swerve sweetener
- ½ tsp vanilla extract

How to Prepare:

1. Beat ½ cup cream in a medium bowl with a hand mixer until it forms peaks.
2. Beat cream cheese with peanut butter in another bowl until creamy.

3. Stir in vanilla, a pinch of salt, and sweetener to the peanut butter mix and combine until smooth.
4. Fold in the prepared whipped cream and mix well until fully incorporated.
5. Divide the mousse into 4 serving glasses.
6. Garnish as desired.
7. Enjoy.

Prep Time: 5 minutes

Servings: 4

Nutritional Values:
- *Calories 290*
- *Total Fat 21.5 g*
- *Saturated Fat 15.2 g*
- *Cholesterol 12.1 mg*
- *Sodium 9 mg*
- *Total Carbs 6.5 g*
- *Sugar 1.2 g*
- *Fiber 0.4 g*
- *Protein 6.2 g*

Cookie Ice Cream

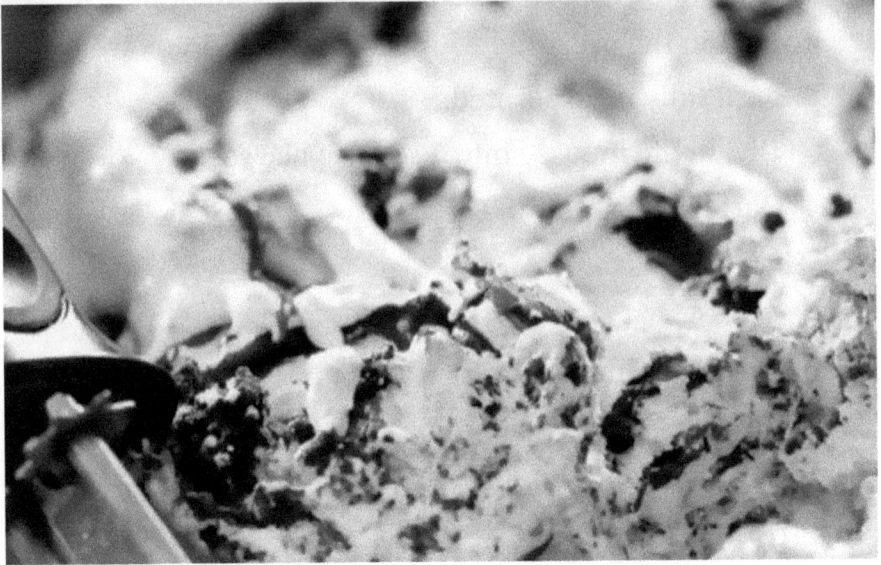

Note: this recipe calls for an ice cream machine

Ingredients:

Cookie Crumbs

- ¾ cup almond flour
- ¼ cup cocoa powder
- ¼ tsp baking soda
- ¼ cup erythritol
- ½ tsp vanilla extract
- 1 ½ tbsp coconut oil, softened
- 1 large egg, room temperature
- Pinch of salt

Ice Cream

- 2 ½ cups whipping cream
- 1 tbsp vanilla extract
- ½ cup erythritol
- ½ cup almond milk, unsweetened

How to Prepare:

1. Preheat your oven at 300 degrees F and layer a 9-inch baking pan with wax paper.
2. Whisk almond flour with baking soda, cocoa powder, salt, and erythritol in a medium bowl.
3. Stir in coconut oil and vanilla extract then mix well until crumbly.
4. Whisk in egg and mix well to form the dough.
5. Spread this dough in the prepared pan and bake for 20 minutes in the preheated oven.
6. Allow the crust to cool then crush it finely into crumbles.
7. Beat cream in a large bowl with a hand mixer until it forms a stiff peak.
8. Stir in erythritol and vanilla extract then mix well until fully incorporated.
9. Pour in milk and blend well until smooth.
10. Add this mixture to an ice cream machine and churn as per the machine's instructions.

11. Add cookie crumbles to the ice cream in the machine and churn again.
12. Place the ice cream in a sealable container and freeze for 2 hours.
13. Scoop out the ice cream and serve.
14. Enjoy.

Prep Time: 5 minutes
Cooking Time: 2 hours
Total Time: 2 hours & 5 minutes
Servings: 2

Nutritional Values:

- *Calories 214*
- *Total Fat 19 g*
- *Saturated Fat 5.8 g*
- *Cholesterol 15 mg*
- *Sodium 123 mg*
- *Total Carbs 6.5 g*
- *Sugar 1.9 g*
- *Fiber 2.1 g*
- *Protein 6.5 g*

Chocolate Avocado Ice Cream

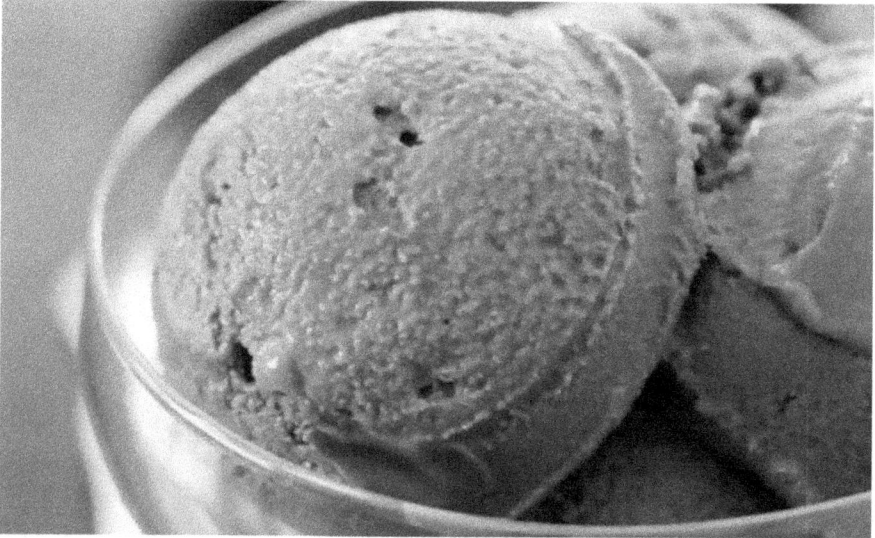

Note: this recipe calls for an ice cream machine

Ingredients:

- 2 large Hass avocados, flesh only
- 1 cup coconut milk
- ½ cup heavy whipping cream
- ½ cup unsweetened cocoa powder
- 2 tsp vanilla extract
- ½ cup erythritol, powdered
- 25 drops liquid stevia
- 6 squares unsweetened Baker's chocolate, chopped

How to Prepare:

1. Mash avocado flesh in a bowl then add coconut milk, vanilla extract, and heavy cream.

2. Beat this mixture with an immersion blender (or another hand mixer) until smooth and creamy.
3. Stir in erythritol, cocoa powder, and stevia and mix well until fully incorporated.
4. Fold in chopped chocolate and mix well gently.
5. Refrigerate the avocado mixture for 12 hours.
6. Churn the ice cream mixture in an ice cream machine as per the machine's instructions.
7. Freeze it for 2 to 4 hours until it hardens.
8. Serve.

Prep Time: 5 minutes
Cooking Time: 16 hours
Total Time: 16 hours & 5 minutes
Servings: 6

Nutritional Values:
- *Calories 282*
- *Total Fat 25.1 g*
- *Saturated Fat 8.8 g*
- *Cholesterol 100 mg*
- *Sodium 117 mg*
- *Total Carbs 9.4 g*
- *Sugar 0.7 g*
- *Fiber 3.2 g*
- *Protein 8 g*

Pumpkin Pecan Ice Cream

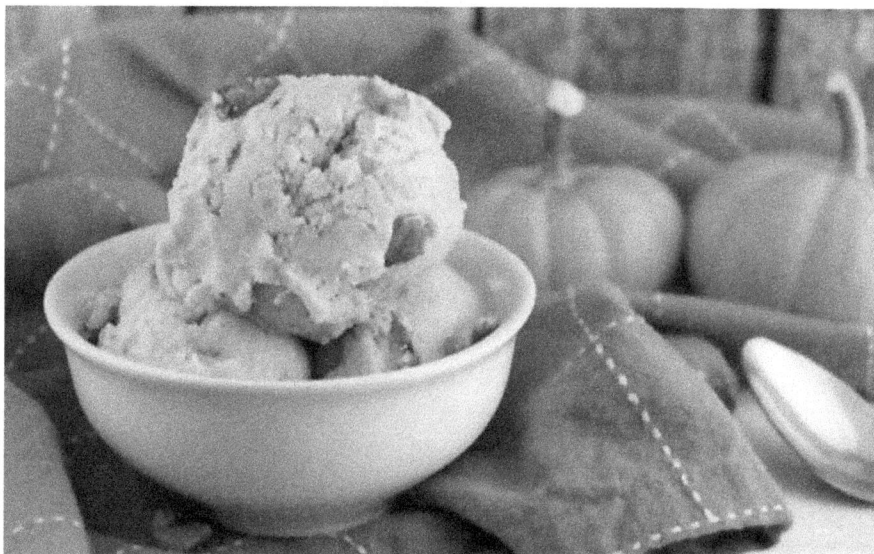

Note: this recipe calls for an ice cream machine

Ingredients:
- ½ cup cottage cheese
- ½ cup pumpkin puree
- 1 tsp pumpkin spice
- 2 cups unsweetened coconut milk
- ½ tsp xanthan gum
- 3 large egg yolks
- 1/3 cup erythritol
- 20 drops liquid stevia
- 1 tsp maple extract
- ½ cup chopped pecans, toasted
- 2 tbsp salted butter

How to Prepare:

1. Add butter to a saucepan and place it over low heat until butter turns brown.
2. Whisk the remaining ingredients in a separate bowl using a hand mixer.
3. Churn this mixture in the ice cream mixture as per the machine's instructions.
4. Toss pecans with butter then add them to the ice cream.
5. Churn again then freeze for 4 hours.
6. Enjoy.

Prep Time: 5 minutes
Cooking Time: 4 hours
Total Time: 4 hours & 5 minutes
Servings: 4

Nutritional Values:

- *Calories 331*
- *Total Fat 38.5 g*
- *Saturated Fat 19.2 g*
- *Cholesterol 141 mg*
- *Sodium 283 mg*
- *Total Carbs 9.2 g*
- *Sugar 3 g*
- *Fiber 1 g*
- *Protein 2.1 g*

Mocha Ice Cream

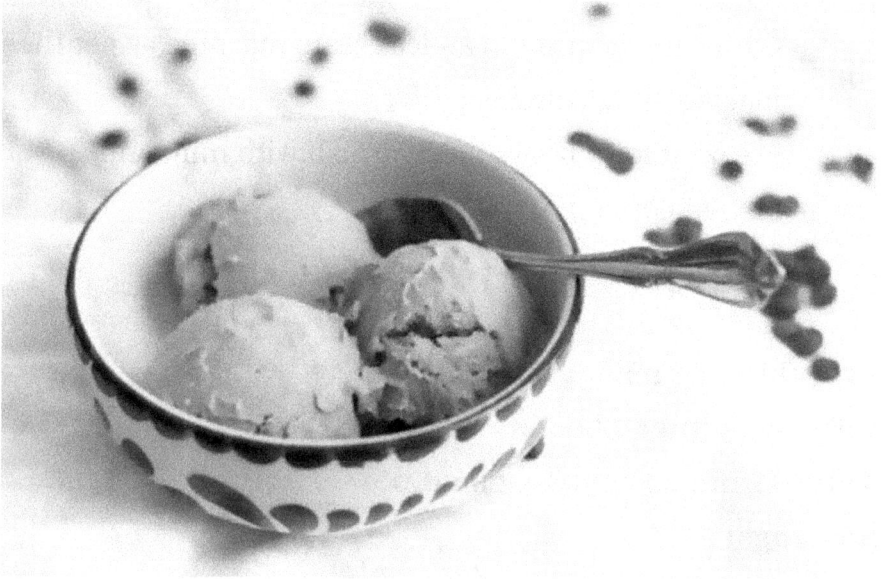

Note: this recipe calls for an ice cream machine

Ingredients:

- 1 cup coconut milk
- ¼ cup heavy whipping cream
- 2 tbsp erythritol
- 15 drops liquid stevia
- 2 tbsp unsweetened cocoa powder
- 1 tbsp instant coffee
- ¼ tsp xanthan gum

How to Prepare:

1. Whisk everything except xanthan gum in a bowl using a hand mixer.

2. Slowly add xanthan gum and stir well to make a thick mixture.
3. Churn the mixture in an ice cream machine as per the machine's instructions.
4. Freeze it for 2 hours then garnish with mint and instant coffee.
5. Serve.

Prep Time: 5 minutes
Cooking Time: 2 hours
Total Time: 2 hours & 5 minutes
Servings: 2

Nutritional Values:
- *Calories 267*
- *Total Fat 44.5 g*
- *Saturated Fat 17.4 g*
- *Cholesterol 153 mg*
- *Sodium 217 mg*
- *Total Carbs 8.4 g*
- *Sugar 2.3 g*
- *Fiber 1.3 g*
- *Protein 3.1 g*

Strawberry Ice Cream

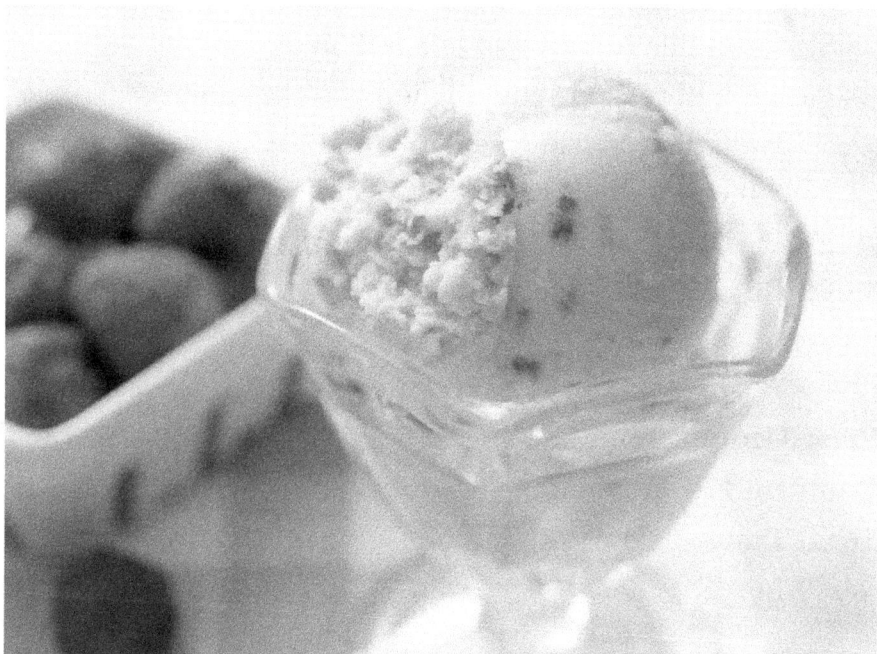

Note: this recipe calls for an ice cream machine

Ingredients:
- 1 cup heavy whipping cream
- 1/3 cup erythritol
- 3 large egg yolks
- ½ tsp vanilla extract
- 1/8 tsp xanthan gum
- 1 tbsp vodka
- 1 cup strawberries, pureed

How to Prepare:
1. Add cream to a pot and place it over low heat and warm it up.

2. Stir in 1/3 cup erythritol and mix well to dissolve.
3. Beat in egg yolks and continue whisking until fluffy.
4. Stir in vanilla extract and mix well until smooth.
5. Lastly, add 1/8 tsp xanthan gum and the vodka.
6. Mix well then transfer the mixture to an ice cream machine and churn as per the machine's instructions.
7. Freeze it for 1 hour then add pureed strawberries.
8. Churn again and freeze for another 1 hour.
9. Serve.

Prep Time: 5 minutes
Cooking Time: 2 hours
Total Time: 2 hours & 5 minutes
Servings: 6

Nutritional Values:
- *Calories 259*
- *Total Fat 34 g*
- *Saturated Fat 10.3 g*
- *Cholesterol 112 mg*
- *Sodium 92 mg*
- *Total Carbs 8.5 g*
- *Sugar 2 g*
- *Fiber 1.3 g*
- *Protein 7.5 g*

Keto Vanilla Ice Cream

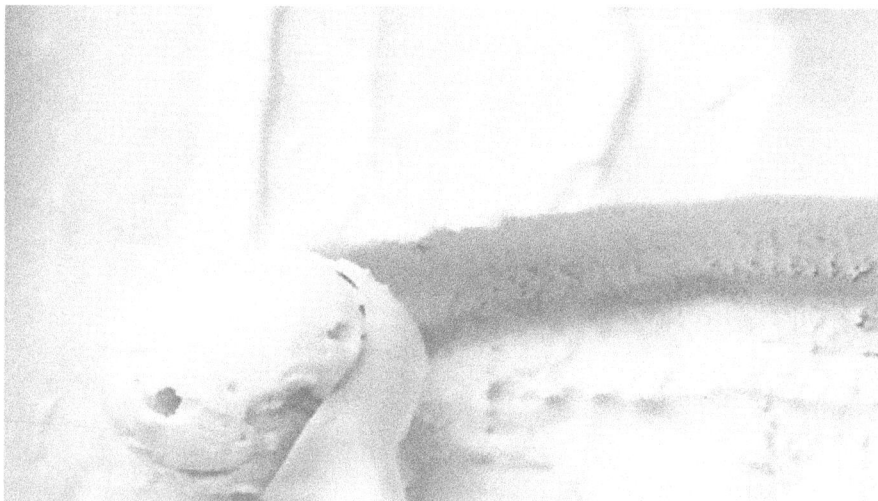

Ingredients:

- 2 15-oz cans coconut milk
- 2 cup heavy cream
- ¼ cup Swerve confectioner's sweetener
- 1 tsp pure vanilla extract
- Pinch kosher salt

How to Prepare:

1. Refrigerate coconut milk for 3 hours or overnight and remove the cream from the top while leaving the liquid in the can. Place the cream in a bowl.
2. Beat the coconut cream using a hand mixer until it forms peaks.

3. Stir in vanilla, sweeteners, and whipped cream then beat well until fluffy.
4. Freeze this mixture for 5 hours.
5. Enjoy.

Prep Time: 8 hours & 5 minutes
Cooking Time: 0 minutes
Total Time: 8 hours & 5 minutes
Servings: 8

Nutritional Values:

- *Calories 255*
- *Total Fat 23.4 g*
- *Saturated Fat 11.7 g*
- *Cholesterol 135 mg*
- *Sodium 112 mg*
- *Total Carbs 2.5 g*
- *Sugar 12.5 g*
- *Fiber 1 g*
- *Protein 7.9 g*

Butter Pecan Ice Cream

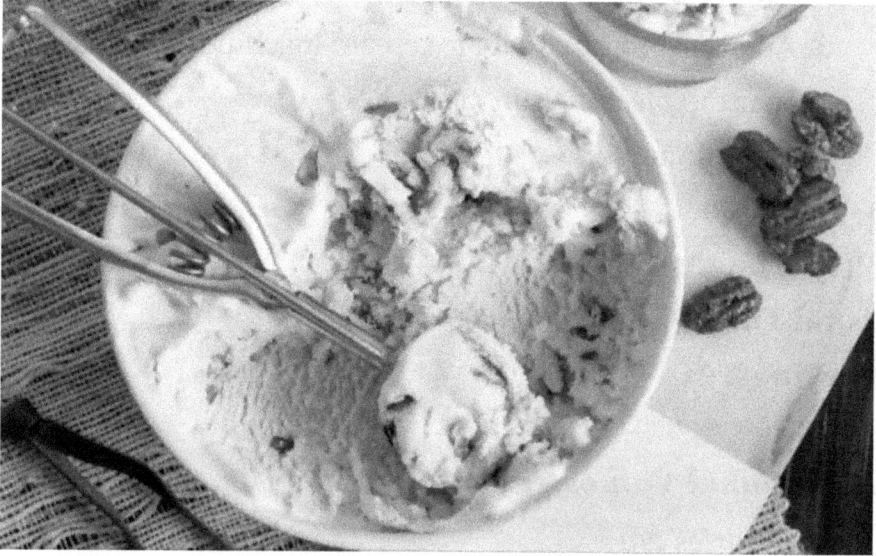

Ingredients:

- 1 ½ cups unsweetened coconut milk
- ¼ cup heavy whipping cream
- 5 tbsp butter
- ¼ cup crushed pecans
- 25 drops liquid stevia
- ¼ tsp xanthan gum

How to Prepare:

1. Place a pan over medium-low heat and melt butter in it until it turns brown.
2. Mix this butter with chopped pecans, heavy cream, and stevia in a bowl.

3. Stir in coconut milk then xanthan gum and mix well until fluffy.
4. Add this mixture to an ice cream machine and churn as per the machine's instructions.
5. Once done, serve.

Prep Time: 5 minutes
Total Time: 5 minutes
Servings: 3

Nutritional Values:

- *Calories 251*
- *Total Fat 24.5 g*
- *Saturated Fat 14.7 g*
- *Cholesterol 165 mg*
- *Sodium 142 mg*
- *Total Carbs 4.3 g*
- *Sugar 0.5 g*
- *Fiber 1 g*
- *Protein 5.9 g*

Conclusion

Baking a delicious and healthy ketogenic meal is all a matter of understanding how to substitute in the right ingredients for the unhealthy ones. Once you understand the basics of all the techniques here you can cook all sorts of keto desserts right at home.

This cookbook can be a mini guide to let you grasp all the necessary information about the ketogenic diet, the role of sugar substitutes, their use, and the ketogenic flours. With different recipes for bread, muffins, buns, snacks, bars, fat bombs, ice cream, and mousses, you have everything you need as a keto-newbie to bake delectable sweet treats in your home.

CPSIA information can be obtained
at www.ICGtesting.com
Printed in the USA
BVHW040213220920
589354BV00014B/912